T0319444

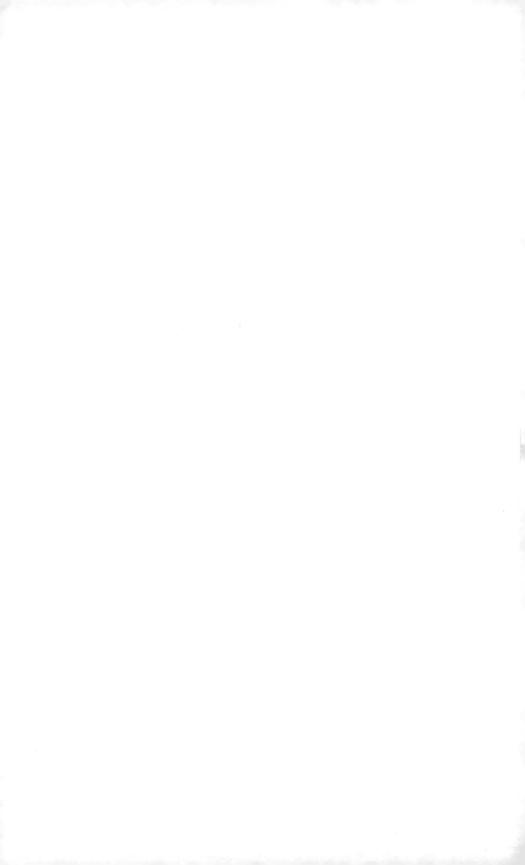

THE STIGMA EFFECT

PATRICK W. CORRIGAN

THE STIGMA EFFECT

Unintended Consequences of Mental
Health Campaigns

Columbia University Press / New York

Columbia University Press
Publishers Since 1893
New York   Chichester, West Sussex
cup.columbia.edu
Copyright © 2018 Columbia University Press
All rights reserved

Library of Congress Cataloging-in-Publication Data
Names: Corrigan, Patrick W., author.
Title: The stigma effect : unintended consequences of mental health
campaigns / Patrick W. Corrigan.
Description: New York : Columbia University Press, [2018] |
Includes bibliographical references and index.
Identifiers: LCCN 2018004624| ISBN 9780231183567 (hardback : alk. paper) |
ISBN 9780231183574 (pbk. : alk. paper) | ISBN 9780231545006 (e-book)
Subjects: | MESH: Mental Disorders—psychology | Social Stigma | Mentally Ill
Persons—psychology | Health Knowledge, Attitudes, Practice
Classification: LCC RC455 | NLM WM 140 | DDC 362.196/89—dc23
LC record available at https://lccn.loc.gov/2018004624

Columbia University Press books are printed on permanent
and durable acid-free paper.

Printed in the United States of America

Cover design: Milenda Nan Ok Lee
Cover art: andersboman © istockphoto / Getty Images

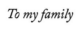

To my family

CONTENTS

ACKNOWLEDGMENTS

T HIS BOOK REPRESENTS more than thirty years with important friends, colleagues, and partners. Those interactions are integral to the ideas herein. My career serving people with serious mental illness started at the *First Step Program* of Niles Township Sheltered Workshop (NTSW) with Jim Stavish, Helene Lome, Ruth Davies-Farmer, and Melinda Stolley. I left there for training at UCLA with Michael Green, Chuck Wallace, and Bob Liberman. Bob has had the singular greatest influence on my career, teaching me that to be a scientist you have to be scholar and entrepreneur. From there I went to the University of Chicago (UC) and was mentored by Bennett Leventhal. I worked at UC as director of its Center for Psychiatric Rehabilitation with Paul Holmes, Barbara Blaser, Rena Moore, Sara Gill, Marie Palmer, Kelvin Oliver, Jon Larson, Amy Watson, Sara Diwan, Bob Lundin, Princess Williams, and Stan McCracken. Stan continues to be my Tai Chi master. Chow Lam and David Penn were important colleagues helping me to better understand disabilities during these years. While at UC, my work evolved from addressing psychiatric disabilities to diminishing psychiatric stigma. This started with a grant from the National Institute of Mental Health to establish the Chicago Consortium on Stigma Research (CCSR) with Mark Heyrman from the UC Law School. CCSR also included Ken Rasinski, Galen Bodenhausen, Vic Ottati, Len Newman, Fred Markowitz, and Beth Angel.

I came to the Illinois Institute of Technology (IIT) in 2005 through the divine intervention of Chow Lam. While at IIT, my work has grown through the influence of Frank Lane, EJ Lee, Jon Larson, Nikki Ditchman, Kelly Kazukaukas, Scott Morris, Ron Landis, Mike Young, and Chris Himes. I am now director of the National Consortium on Stigma and Empowerment (NCSE) with IIT colleagues Lindsay Sheehan and Jon Larson. Lindsay is my right arm in NCSE's work. I have enjoyed stimulating discussions with several students including Kristin Kosyluk, Patrick Michaels, Katherine Nieweglowski, Binoy Shah, Sang Qin, and Maya Al-Khouja. My work has blossomed through the partnership with Sue Pickett from Advocates for Human Potential. I am privileged to work with health providers from Trilogy, Thresholds, and Heartland Health Outreach. Thanks to my research team including Sonya Ballentine, Ali Torres, Lorena Lara, Janis Sayer, Annie Schmidt, Deysi Paniagua, Dana Kraus, and Cheryl Wan. Special thanks to Katherine Nieweglowski and Maggie Carson for yeoman's work helping me polish this manuscript.

My work on stigma is influenced by a slew of ongoing relationships with outstanding scholars including Bruce Link (the father of modern stigma research), Bernice Pescosolido, Otto Wahl, Jo Phelan, Phil Yanos, David Roe, Paul Lysaker, Heather Stuart, Graham Thornicroft, Norman Sartorius, Jen Ohan, Kirsten Cathoor, Luca Pingani, Michelle Salyers, Hector Tsang, Anthony Jorm, Stephen Hinshaw, Winnie Mak, Sara Evans-Lacko, Shirli Werner, Rebecca Palpant Shimketts, Mike Pietrus, Georg Schomerus, Matthias Angermeyer, Katrina Scior, Eillis Hennessey, Carolyn Heary, Peter Byrne, Rebecca Puhl, and Perla Werner. Most important among these is my student and now dear colleague, Nicolas Rüsch at the University of Ulm. Nicolas has been an essential partner with me for almost twenty years.

Stigma is only resolved by people who have been harmed by its poison. Several with lived experienced have been mentors and friends including Sally Clay, Ruth Ralph, Bob Lundin, Sally Zinman, Jay Mahler, Keris Myrick, Keith Mahar, Ingrid Ozols, Khatera Aslami, Eduardo Vega, and Jennifer Brown. *Honest Open Proud* is the mainstay of my current work in erasing stigma. HOP partners have included Suzette Urbashich, Sue McKenzie, Michelle Andra, Dan O'Brien-Mazza, Dinesh Mittal, David Smelson, Nynke Mulder, and Chris White.

Much of this book represents a personal journey. Thanks to Rob McSay, a psychiatrist, friend, and savior. Thanks to Jon and Stan for being there during hard times. Most of all, my ideas and success are due to family. Only recently have I looked back to understand challenges I wrought on loved ones. My wife, Georgeen Carson, is the single fact of my continued presence with any semblance of impact. Georgeen also taught me about living with social justice in the world; she was a Cook County Public Defender for more than thirty years, providing legal assistance to Chicagoans no matter what their crime. I am pleased to say that Georgeen and I were able to pass this priority to our children. Abe is now a paralegal in a Chicago law firm specializing in righting civil injustice. Liz worked for the American Red Cross in Washington, D.C., and is on her way as a Peace Corps volunteer in Tanzania.

PREFACE

Progressives charge into battle wherever injustice occurs. Stigma is one such injustice that plagues the twenty-first century. Progressives often err in writing these wrongs. This is the *stigma effect*. This book addresses the stigma of mental illness, campaigns gone awry, and approaches shown to be effective. Central to these strategies are anti-stigma programs led by people with lived experience of the stigmatized condition.

THE TWENTIETH AND TWENTY-FIRST CENTURIES are hailed as times of progress and success. Significant health challenges have been overcome. Technology eased life, allowing drudgeries to be replaced by fulfillment. Democracy lessened the tyranny of oppressors. Compared to the Middle Ages, enlightenment has been realized, but clearly not for everyone. Out-groups defined by ethnicity, religion, gender, sexual orientation, and health conditions fail to enjoy these advances. Social injustices crush the victories of the past two centuries. These injustices are essential motivators to right our societies. Progressives do so with energy and optimism, seeking to replace prejudice and discrimination with opportunity and self-determination. Sometimes we are victorious, adding to the masses who are able to enjoy our successes. Gains in civil rights and women's suffrage have addressed the social injustices faced by African Americans and women to a significant extent. Sometimes we stumble; big steps fail to bring lasting solutions. Racism remains a virulent force. Sometimes we blunder. Some progressive efforts not only fall short but actually backfire. Consider three examples.

In the 1960s, progressives sought to address racism by promoting color blindness, the idea that ethnic differences do not matter, that we are all the same. Hence, we should ignore values that define the differences. Blacks, for example, were asked to ignore their cultural roots. Although the goal was to stifle ethnic disparity, it more likely promoted white priorities. The Black Power movement arose to reaffirm the importance of African American identity. Among its many meanings, Black Power symbolized African American efforts at rediscovery and self-determination. This included recognition of African culture, history, and accomplishments with pride. It sometimes included a call for Black Nationalism, which threatened many whites, a seemingly unexpected result of color-blind proponents who naively assumed we could come together under one neutral tent.

Consider another example. In the 1990s, President Bill Clinton dealt with homophobia in the military by supporting Don't Ask, Don't Tell (DADT) policies. Prior to then, the military actively sought to ban gays and lesbians from service. DADT made it unlawful for military branches to exclude people because of sexual orientation. In return, DADT barred gay and lesbian personnel from "openly" enlisting or remaining in military service. Gay enlistees and officers were precluded from talking about their orientation. Although an improvement over previous policies, DADT encouraged service men and women to be closeted by allowing them to stay in the military as long as they hid essential parts of their identity. DADT soon encountered significant resistance. It was repugnant to progressives, who believed that being out and open about one's sexual orientation were fundamental to an esteemed life, everywhere, including the military. The Log Cabin Republicans, the nation's largest Republican gay organization, challenged DADT's constitutionality by arguing that it violated the rights of gay military members to free speech, due process, and open association. After several years of debate, DADT was repealed during the Obama Administration in 2010.

A third example, which is personally important to me as a Jesuit-trained Catholic, was Pope Francis's inaugural mass on March 19, 2013. Jorge Bergoglio chose Francis as his regnal name in homage to St. Francis, the thirteenth century friar renowned for preachings related to care for the poor. In this light, the Pope quoted during his inauguration verse 25:40 from

Matthew's gospel where Christ said to his apostles, "Whatsoever you do to the **least** of my brethren that you do unto me." While clearly seeking to motivate the masses toward accepting responsibility for all one's brothers and sisters, the quote repeats an unintended stigma; namely, that a person who is disadvantaged is somehow less than others. It perpetuates a dated notion of charity—that the haves *bestow* upon the have nots their advantages. The rich give to the poor, the educated to the uneducated, the healthy to the sick. This promotes a one-up hierarchy in which the former are somehow better than the latter. Current approaches to social justice replace notions of "alms to the poor" with those of empowerment and rightful opportunity for all. Social justice is achieved when everyone is empowered to pursue a life that fulfills personal goals.

I do not believe that Pope Francis sought to disempower or otherwise debase people with fewer advantages. Quite the contrary; his efforts to return the church to concerns of common people is remarkable. Similarly, I do not believe that purveyors of color blindness or DADT were trying to worsen the lot of people of color or the lesbian, gay, bisexual, transgender, questioning (LGBTQ) community. But, indeed, that's what they did. Advocates against social injustice need to learn from such mistaken intentions to craft ever-better approaches toward empowerment and self-determination.

The focus of this book is on the social injustices experienced by people with behavioral health challenges: mental illness and substance use disorders. Research clearly shows that stigma of mental illness can be as disabling as illness symptoms and dysfunctions. In the past ten to fifteen years, recognition of the egregious effects of stigma has led to large and organized efforts to erase its effects through national policies, privately organized social-marketing campaigns, and grassroots advocacy. At the same time, research efforts meant to describe stigma's effects and evaluate anti-stigma interventions have boomed. As a result, communities of "stigma busters" have begun to identify ways that might erase stigma's harm. But in some cases, these well-meant interventions not only yield little benefit but seem to worsen stigma.

- Education, especially of adults, about the myths and facts of mental illness may yield little benefit, instead adding to misconceptions about psychiatric disorder.

- Campaigns to decrease stigma in order to get people into treatment—by, for example, framing depression as a treatable illness—might worsen stigmatizing notions of difference—"that the diseased person is unlike me"—which exacerbates prejudice and discrimination.
- Broad-based population campaigns using social, entertainment, and news media may be less cost-effective than local, grassroots campaigns.

A focus on the stigma effect—the unintended consequences of anti-stigma efforts—has several benefits. Advocates of all stripes need to understand what fails to work, especially when evidence contradicts preferred perspectives. For example, many advocates in the Western world believe that social problems can be educated away; teach the facts, and biases will disappear. Such beliefs need to be greeted with caution. Through these cautions, broader and deeper understandings of stigma and stigma change emerge. I believe that the stigma against people with mental illness is in the same category as racism, sexism, ageism, and homophobia. Hence, solutions should rest solely in the agendas of people with lived experience harmed by these stigmas. Programs that lead to enduring and meaningful success will emerge in the light of ongoing cautious appraisal of their efforts.

Progressives sometimes approach stigma change uncritically. Because it is an injustice, advocates think, "What's there to know?" Stigma is wrong. Together advocates can quash it. One goal of this book is to learn from unintended consequences so advocates are better equipped to change stigma meaningfully.

THREE PERSPECTIVES

I write this book from three personal perspectives: science, advocacy, and personal experience. I am firstly a *scientist* believing that careful research will significantly advance understanding of the harmful effects of stigma as well as effective ways to tackle it. My first pursuits were in experimental psychopathology trying to explain the social and coping skills deficits among people with schizophrenia in terms of neuropsychological dysfunctions related to attention, memory, and executive functioning. This basic work dovetailed with a burgeoning portfolio of studies on psychiatric rehabilitation, the collection of interventions meant to help people with serious mental illness achieve personal goals related to education, work, independent living, and relationships. I did this work as a provider of mental health services. I have been licensed as a clinical psychologist for more than twenty-five years, at one time directing an "aftercare" program for people with serious mental illness at the University of Chicago, Department of Psychiatry. I directed this program for fourteen years, with the program logging more than 20,000 service hours per year.

The most meaningful research comes from personal experience. While running the aftercare service, I observed how program participants learned to manage symptoms and dysfunctions so they were ready to achieve their goals in the community. They were ready to get a job or live on their own. Unfortunately, their goals were often crushed by the community they sought to reenter. Employers did not want to hire people with serious mental illness. Landlords did not want to rent to them. Barriers to recovery did not reside in the person, but in the community in which he or she resided. This is what I discovered to be stigma.

At the time (about 1998), research was limited to the esteemed work of Bruce Link at Columbia University and a few others. So I consumed this literature, as well as more basic research from social psychology and sociology, to develop a basic comprehension of the effects of stigma on people with lived experience. I then organized a group of like-minded scholars at the University of Chicago and launched the Chicago Consortium on Stigma Research (CCSR) with funding from the National Institute of Mental Health. Since then, CCSR evolved into the National Consortium on Stigma and Empowerment, with partners at more than twenty academic programs and ten advocacy groups around the world. We have been continuously funded by the National Institutes of Health during that time, generating well over 200 peer-reviewed papers as well as a dozen books. In 2015, I began a two-year tenure on the Committee on the Science of Changing Behavioral Health Social Norms of the National Academy of Sciences (NAS). Our subsequent report summarized the state of the science in order to guide U.S. efforts for a nationwide anti-stigma program (National Academies Press, 2016). Last year, I became inaugural editor of *Stigma and Health*, a journal of the American Psychological Association.

Stigma and Health gives me a ringside seat in following innovative research. I use the research summarized in the NAS report, as well as findings from the literature at large, to reinforce claims made about stigma and stigma change herein, perhaps with an ego-blinded bias toward the 100+ peer-reviewed studies achieved by our research group.

Despite the positivism of science, I am skeptical of the possibilities that come out of research alone. Where was the scientist when Martin Luther King Jr., eloquently addressed civil rights? Did Susan B. Anthony consult with demographers when planning her actions to promote women's suffrage? I realized that the effects of my work would only be meaningful by assuming a progressive approach to the social injustices experienced by people with serious mental illness. Hence, I am secondly an *advocate* striving to make real world changes in the lives of people with mental illness. Tackling social injustice is valuable for me partly because it represents the sincere results of a Catholic education (from kindergarten to bachelor's degree) steeped in Matthew's gospel. It also reflects the historical times of my childhood. I am a 1960s voyeur; I was too young to actually participate in the protests but felt inspired by those tactics to make real-world change. In the past decade, I realized I had to be in the midst of the stigma fray if my research was to make a difference. Hence, my studies are governed by the advocate's imperative. Just as clinical research is valued by the degree to which it betters treatments for people with mental illness, so stigma research is important when it leads to better stigma change. I have learned more from peers and advocates with lived experience about stigma and stigma change than I have from any collection of scholarly papers.

I am thirdly a *person* with lived experience of serious mental illness. The challenges of serious mental illness have plagued me for more than forty years: symptoms, emergencies, failures, meds, and hospitalization. Stigma is neither solely an object of my study nor just an abstraction. I know the shame of having to drop out of school because of overwhelming panic; the guilt of having to explain to my children what I was doing in the hospital; and the worry that I will fail again. To be clear, many of my challenges arose from the disabling effects of symptoms and dysfunctions. However, the course of my mental health experiences was worsened by having to deal with the world around me, and its messages of disapproval, shame, and secrecy.

I use all three perspectives in authoring this book. I believe mental illness and its stigma is a phenomenon that can be understood and impacted using the methods of behavioral science. I also believe, however, that the power of research can only be valued by its real-world impact. Hence, the science is explicitly governed by the advocate's agenda. I cannot escape my own lived experience herein and ways it colored my perspective on stigma. Hence, I share stories from my personal life that illustrate key points. Almost all my writing to date has been for professional audiences where journal guidelines discourage the first-person voice, thereby promoting a sense of the objectivity science means to stoke. Most of my twenty-five-year history has avoided using pronouns such as I, my, and mine; you could read 400 page texts with first-person voice entirely absent. However, the third perspective of this book yearned for a different writing style, in part because of personal perspectives that recur throughout. The book includes textboxes that provide first-person perspective on key issues related to stigma and stigma change. The "I" is evident, admittedly a difficult task for which I beg the readers' indulgence.

A WORD ABOUT LANGUAGE

Words we use to refer to people with mental health challenges and stigma are loaded and, therefore, an important focus for people attempting to impact stigma. This issue is of such importance that it is the focus of chapter 4. Here, though, I define how the central object of the book, the person harmed by stigma, is referenced. Mostly, I favor person-first language broadly endorsed by health and disabilities advocates: "people with lived experience." Person first conveys the idea that people are more than the experience of mental illness. They are not reduced to schizophrenics, or manics, or depressives. It also focuses on lived experience that defines the person's class. They are not a group specified by psychiatric diagnoses but rather described by a set of shared experiences related to mental health challenges, community reactions, and treatments.

Still, I will occasionally reference people as patients. Patient refers to the essential role people have within a health care system, a central role in their lived experience, leading to being victimized by stigma. *Patient* is a loaded word to be sure. It refers to an object of care in a one-down relationship with treatment providers. But sometimes, this reference is essential to points I make herein. It is as receiver of mental health services that particular discussions make sense. By the way, while words like *patient* might suggest disempowerment and disapproval, as a hypothesis, this assumption has not been supported by research. Surveys of people with lived experience have not been able to find any one label—patient, client, consumer, user, person—as more or less satisfactory than others (Mueser, Glynn, Corrigan, & Baber, 1996; Penn & Nowlin-Drummond, 2001). That said, I still encourage readers to be sensitive to issues of language as they choose to venture into concerns about mental illness stigma.

A book limited to analyzing failures would be unsatisfying indeed if that is where the discussion ends. Ending social injustice, and not simply describing it, is the ultimate goal. Hence, the book ends with discussion of what research suggests may be potent approaches to stigma change. Once again, I admit biases that influenced my research. Just as approaches to racism, sexism, and ageism must be led by people who are harmed by these injustices—people of color, women, and older adults—so must approaches to erasing the stigma of mental illness be owned and led by people with mental health challenges. I am a white, male, Irish American who is hugely motivated to resolve racism and sexism. But I relegate my role to the back seat of efforts to right these inequities. In that light, people with lived experience need to be driving efforts meant to correct the stigma of mental illness. This leaves other advocates in unexpected roles. Psychiatrists, psychologists, family members, and mental health system administrators who have keen interest in resolving mental health stigma need to accept their support role in tackling stigma. Whites cannot speak for blacks in rectifying racism. Psychiatrists cannot do this for people with lived experience. Ultimately, the pernicious effects of stigma are resolved when replaced by beliefs and behaviors that empower people with mental illness.

THE STIGMA EFFECT

1

WHO IS THE PERSON WITH SERIOUS MENTAL ILLNESS?

S TIGMA IS A social construction, not a fact. Societal beliefs and values lead to misguided and hurtful stigma about a group. Sometimes these beliefs emerge from what science has to say about how the research describes mental illness. I do not imply that contemporary knowledge about mental illness is meant to be stigmatizing. But, the body of information may set the frame in which stigmatizing beliefs evolve. Therefore, the place to begin is how contemporary science has come to describe the person with mental illness. Many ideas have led to advancements in services for people struggling with their illnesses. Others have fanned the flames of stigma. They exacerbate the stigma effect.

In the last fifty years, medical and social scientists have made notable strides in understanding and treating serious mental illnesses.[1] Yet during this time we have also made major missteps in the way we characterize people with mental illness, often leading to damaging stereotypes and ineffective, or even harmful, standards of care. "People with serious mental illnesses are incapable of enjoying good jobs, independent living, and intimate relationships. They are potentially dangerous, and likely to harm others. Patients[2]

---

1. The terms *mental illness* and *psychiatric disorder* are used interchangeably throughout the text.
2. As said in the preface, words are important when considering stigma and *patient* is sometimes seen as one such word. I use different terms throughout the book to refer to people with "lived experience" to represent their role or relationship to the discussion topic. I use *patient* or *client*, in particular, when issues being discussed reflect a person's relationship with a service provider.

need ongoing supervision from health care professionals to help them avoid life-threatening decisions." Although these may sound like uninformed statements from an ignorant public, they actually represent professional philosophies that were once largely accepted by experts in mental health.

This is not meant as an indictment of the sciences of psychology and psychiatry. Many critics see the "medical model" as an example of what is wrong with mental health research and practice. The medical model is a perspective of health driven largely by basic biological and medical sciences, which, in some forms, may reduce mental health challenges to the sum of symptoms and brain chemistry. In the 1960s, these objections coalesced into the antipsychiatry movement, a coordinated coalition of ex-patients who recognized the harm of medical approaches and demanded that the mental health care system be reformed. The movement's power came from grassroots groups such as the Mental Patient's Liberation Front in Boston and Insane Liberation Front of Portland, Oregon. Scholars including Thomas Szasz (a psychiatrist who wrote *The Myth of Mental Illness*) and Michel Foucault (a social philosopher who authored *Madness and Civilization: A History of Insanity in the Age of Reason*) provided an intellectual voice for the movement. Yet the truly eloquent spokespeople were ex-patients, such as Howard "Howie the Harp" Geld:

> I've been diagnosed as a schizophrenic, as psychotic, as manic-depressive and as psychotic depressive. I don't really believe in those labels, but there have been times in my life when I went into what can be called a manic episode, and when I went into severe depressions. What I'm doing with my life right now is trying to learn how to control what I call manic energy. If it can be controlled and directed and channeled, it could be really valuable and real powerful. I'd rather learn how to control it, rather than be cured of it.
>
> (Van Gelder, 1995)

Members of the antipsychiatry movement railed against treatments such as psychiatric medication, electroconvulsive therapy (ECT), and inpatient hospitalization, a concern that continues for some mental health advocates today. They frequently viewed themselves as ex-patients and survivors. Survivors did not outlast the illness, they survived the treatment.

Although I am sympathetic with some antipsychiatry concerns, I do not believe the medical enterprise is fundamentally flawed. Quite the contrary—breakthroughs in medicine, surgery, and the allied health professions have led to tremendous advances in health and wellness. I do not hesitate to use these services for myself or my family, including psychiatric services. I become concerned when antipsychiatry proponents dismiss all clinical practices as out of hand, because I believe individuals may, at times, benefit from particular treatments. As a clinical psychologist and a patient, I recognize the benefits of many models of mental illness and of interventions meant to address them.

Nevertheless, I believe that misconceptions about mental illness, which form the basis of many common stigmas, have their basis in psychiatry and psychology. Hence, I have two goals in this chapter. First, I briefly review the state of the science of mental illness, with a special focus on findings that can help those challenged by serious mental illnesses. In the process, I will highlight occasions when scientists posed mistaken suppositions that undermined patients' goals. "People do not recover. The illness will only get worse. They cannot make competent decisions about their lives." Understanding how misconceptions such as these evolved out of the mental health system is an important step in understanding how stigma emerges and grows.

DIAGNOSES OF SERIOUS MENTAL ILLNESS

Psychiatric professionals in the United States and much of the world rely on the *Diagnostic and Statistical Manual of Mental Disorders*, currently in its fifth edition (DSM-5; American Psychiatric Association, 2013) to diagnose and classify mental illness. According to the DSM-5, a psychiatric diagnosis or disorder is a *clinically significant* syndrome that is associated with *distress* or *dysfunction* or with increased risk of death, pain, or loss of freedom. Diagnoses represent a collection of symptoms and dysfunctions that cohere into meaningful psychiatric syndromes. Symptoms are the negative experiences of the illness, such as depression, hallucinations, or panic. Dysfunctions represent the absence of normal functioning: poor social skills, the inability to work, or diminished self-care. Also important is the *course* of the illness. Psychiatric syndromes are not static phenomena but vary among individuals by onset and trajectory. (Course will be discussed later in this chapter.) Professionals may speculate on prognosis, or outcome, based on a patient's diagnosis and course. Four diagnostic syndromes are commonly associated with serious mental illnesses: schizophrenia, mood disorders, anxiety disorders, and personality disorders.

Schizophrenia is the prototypic "serious" mental illness. The narrowest definition is restricted to evidence of delusions or prominent hallucinations, with the patient not having insight into the pathological nature of the hallucinations. A broader definition includes other symptoms such as disorganized speech, grossly disorganized behavior, social withdrawal, apathy, poverty of speech, and flat affect. Schizophrenia is considered a spectrum disorder; there are a variety of disorders that may vary in course and outcome but share similar symptoms and dysfunctions. Other diagnoses in the spectrum include *schizoaffective* and *schizophreniform* disorder. Schizoaffective disorder combines experiences of schizophrenia with recurring major depressive or manic episodes. People with schizophreniform disorder meet the diagnostic criteria for schizophrenia, except that the course of the disease is much shorter (typically between one and six months).

Depression and mania are common examples of *mood disorders*. Symptoms of depression include prominent sadness for prolonged periods or significant *anhedonia* (feeling no enjoyment from any activities, including those that were previously pleasurable). People with major depression also experience *vegetative signs*, significant changes in sleep, appetite, energy, and libido. Interestingly, the changes can either represent an increase or decrease from the person's baseline. For example, people with major depression may report sleeping significantly more or not being able to sleep as much; noticeable weight gain or decreased appetite; and having little energy or experiencing high levels of agitation. Suicidal ideation—thoughts of suicide—is often viewed as a diagnostic indicator of depression.

Mania is marked by a decreased need for sleep, increased talking, often with pressured speech, distractibility, risky behavior, inflated self-esteem, and grandiosity (an unrealistic sense of superiority). People with *bipolar disorder* experience separate periods of major depression and mania interspersed with periods of normal mood. The manic and depressive episodes may last

A Disabling Experience

I've been alternately diagnosed with major depression, bipolar disorder, and anxiety disorder, experiencing symptoms recurrently for more than forty years. Two clusters are prominent: crippling anxiety with panic and all-encompassing depression with a doom-and-gloom view of my future. I can run through all the symptoms from the DSM but most symptoms and diagnoses do not capture "IT." It is episodic with a beginning and an end. I can usually tell when I am in it, often starting with a panic attack from work-related stress. It is a sense of being possessed, not in the delusional sense of spiritual possession but just as all-encompassing and demanding. It greets me every morning of the episode but ebbs through the day. It physically hurts; it is heavy; I can't get a full breath. It colors everything dark. I get tired and, as I age, worry about whether this is another one of those disabling episodes. I become sad and tired of living. It typically persists for a few months to more than two years in the longest case. Only when my professional career evolved into a clinical practice did I understand it disables me. The depth of the disabilities has been difficult to describe. Unlike some people with schizophrenia or major affective disorders, I was never unemployed for long stretches, homeless, or alienated from loved ones. Nonetheless, my experiences were disabling.

My brother, Mike, and I were the first in our extended family to attend college. I graduated with a bachelor's degree in physics from Creighton University in 1978. My life goal was to become a physician in the spirit of my TV heroes—Dr. Kildare and Ben Casey—and I was admitted to Creighton's School of Medicine on a public health service training scholarship. Although I struggled with minor mental health challenges as an undergraduate, my first experience with major mental illness slammed me during my first semester of medical school. I became overwhelmed with the stress of course work, and after a valiant, yearlong try, dropped out. I reframed myself as a wounded hero and aimed for a PhD program in clinical

(continued)

psychology. I was admitted to the program at the Illinois Institute of Technology (IIT) in 1981, panicked during the first week of the program, and dropped out. (Ironically, I went back to IIT in 2005 as psychology faculty.) Panic undoes me, but the resulting sense of worthlessness and hopelessness cements the experience.

I earned a master's degree in a less-demanding clinical psychology program at Roosevelt University two years later, along the way becoming interested in the intersection of philosophy of science and psychological practice. I matriculated to a PhD program at the University of Chicago on the conceptual foundations of science on an NSF fellowship and again, within a week, freaked out and quit. I decided to pursue my PsyD in clinical psychology at the Illinois School of Professional Psychology and after six years was able to graduate with a doctorate. I became an NIMH-supported fellow, working among some of the world leaders on understanding and treating people with serious mental illness. It was a heady time in my life. I had a one-year-old son, was living in Southern California, and felt like I had finally made it. I experienced overwhelming panic during the first months of the program and had to escape. Unlike previous episodes, this time I was able to hold on for a year, seeking to get a job and move on from student life.

I was offered a faculty position at the University of Chicago Department of Psychiatry in the fall of 1990. Within the first week I found myself in a faculty meeting with twenty white-coated colleagues and responded with what, in retrospect, seemed to be a muted form of PTSD. I was back where it all started, in medical school! This time, however, I went to an emergency outpatient clinic and got help. I made plans with my wife, Georgeen, on how to get through one month at a time until my urgent need to bail passed; I remained at UC for fourteen years.

Disabilities are caused by symptoms or dysfunctions that prevent people from achieving life goals and dreams. I repeatedly was unable to pursue vocational goals because anxiety and depression derailed my career for more than ten years, a period of time when my dear wife and friends were becoming lawyers, doctors, and professors. I eventually found my path and ended up in a good place vocationally. I am reminded of a one-liner from Robin Williams that I have used with my students, "I am proof, boys and girls, that you can fuck up and still do well."

weeks or even months. Episodes as short as a few days followed by an episode of opposite polarity are not uncommon.

Anxiety disorders are characterized by extreme worry about current or future events, leading to physical symptoms including rapid heartbeat, shortness of breath, tingling, and panic. Anxiety can manifest as a generalized disorder (e.g., excessive, pervasive, and difficult to control) or in more specific manifestations such as separation anxiety, social phobia, agoraphobia, or phobia of a particular experience (e.g., fear of heights). Many laypeople view anxiety disorders as less severe than schizophrenia and mood disorders. Yet they can be extremely disabling, preventing people from achieving significant life goals.

Personality disorders are characterized by disabling ways in which people relate to and think about their environment and self. Symptoms and dysfunctions include inflexible or otherwise maladaptive manifestations of normal personality traits. Borderline Personality Disorder is often viewed as the most challenging of personality disorders marked by a pervasive pattern of instability in social relationships, self-image, and emotions, exacerbated by severe impulsivity. Impulsive behaviors can include self-mutilation or suicide. Because social relationships are tumultuous, people with borderline personality disorders frequently lack a support network that can help them cope with even small problems. As a result, minor episodes of depression and anxiety can explode into overwhelming stress. People with Borderline Personality Disorder may have significant difficulty accomplishing employment, relationship, and other independent life goals because of these symptoms. Many can greatly benefit from rehabilitation.

SUBSTANCE-RELATED AND ADDICTIVE DISORDERS

Research suggests that almost half of people with serious mental illness struggle with additional challenges due to addictions (Kessler et al., 1996; Kenneson, Funderburk, & Maisto, 2013). Likelihood that a person can meet criteria for alcohol abuse during their lifetime ranges from 13 to 18 percent; drug abuse ranges from 7.7 to 7.9 percent (Merikangas & McClair, 2012). The DSM-5 defines substance-related and addictive disorders in terms of ten classes of drugs: alcohol, caffeine, cannabis, hallucinogens (such as LSD or peyote), inhalants (glue or paint), sedatives (barbiturates or antianxiety medications like valium or Ativan), stimulants (amphetamines or cocaine), opioids (heroin or OxyContin), tobacco, and substances not otherwise classified. Substance use is considered "disordered" when regular use causes cognitive, behavioral, or physiological symptoms that lead to impaired control, social disabilities, or risky use that undermine life goals related to education, work, independent living, relationships, and health. A characteristic irony of substance use disorders is their continued use despite the person realizing harmful effects of the substance.

CHALLENGES OF "DIAGNOSIS"

Although diagnosis is the backbone of the descriptive enterprise, it has conceptual limitations that may worsen stigma: the hunt for pathognomonic symptoms, the reification of diagnosis nomenclature, and the demonstration of disease insight.

PATHOGNOMONIC SYMPTOMS

Pathognomonic symptoms are characteristics unique to specific disorders. This kind of specificity leads to differential diagnoses between seemingly similar disorders; does the person hearing voices have schizophrenia or is she in a manic episode representing bipolar disorder? Diabetes mellitus, for example, has been pathognomonically defined in terms of chronic fasting blood glucose levels. Lymphoma is defined through positive signs in imaging, blood work, and histology. Primary care doctors use these signs to direct patients to specific and effective care.

German psychiatrist Kurt Schneider (1939) defined first-rank symptoms that he believed were pathognomonic of schizophrenia; they included auditory hallucinations, thought withdrawal ("thoughts are being taken out of my head"), thought insertion ("people are putting thoughts into my head"), or thought broadcasting ("people can hear my thoughts"). Subsequent research, however, has been unable to confirm these symptoms as pathognomonic of schizophrenia. In fact, no symptoms have met pathognomonic criteria for any DSM-5 disorder. Think of the implications here. Diagnosis becomes a much more difficult enterprise. Psychiatric professionals do not have tests that unequivocally suggest an individual presents with diagnosis X instead of Y. As a result, psychiatric symptoms are better understood as continuous dimensions rather than black or white characteristics. In fact, there are not symptoms that even distinguish the true seriousness of schizophrenia from more benign disorders like depression.

Consider hallucinations, which one might think are incontrovertible evidence of psychosis. They are not. There are experiences of hypnogogic and hypnopompic hallucinations (auditory and visual experiences that occur as one is falling asleep or waking up) that research shows occurs in almost 40 percent of the population (Ohayon, 2000). Alternatively, many people report corner-of-the-eye experiences that could be misunderstood as hallucinations. "Hey. Was that my dead Aunt Lillian I just saw out of the corner of my eye?" Hence, we need to be cautious about simplistic labels of people and their problems.

REIFYING DIAGNOSIS

Diagnoses are essentially created by scientists as conceptual placeholders meant to hang ideas in order to serve research or clinical agendas. They really do not exist as entities outside conceptual domains. Still, diagnoses do yield benefits. For the researcher, individual diagnoses are the center of a conceptual sphere from which explanatory science radiates. Consider depression. From neuroscience, depression is described by neural transmitters, cerebral tracts, and histology. From phenomenology, depression includes characteristic mood symptoms and vegetative signs. From social science, depression may be understood in terms of poor social skills and individual relationships. Diagnosis also has value as a clinical heuristic.

Applying symptoms that emerge from phenomenology helps the clinician to identify diagnoses relevant to specific patient complaints. Diagnoses implicate strategies that might remedy these complaints.

Trouble arises when diagnoses are believed to be real things that exist outside the conceptual world; this is reification. Problems occur when depression is thought to be a meaningful entity beyond theory, a thing unto itself. Thingness traps researchers, clinicians, and patients alike. The radiating sphere of the depression concept, according to the DSM-5, is defined by a set of inclusion and exclusion criteria. Research that does not fit the criteria may potentially be sorted into another sphere or discarded altogether. Researchers are often comfortable with the squishiness of paradigms so reification may be less problematic for them. The problems increase exponentially for clinicians and patients. Clinicians can fall victim to talking to a person's diagnosis and not the person. "Fran has schizophrenia. I know she wants to go back to work, but she doesn't understand how disabling schizophrenia can be." Reified diagnosis is even worse because of stickiness. Diagnoses are hard to shake. Consider an example. When in practice, I would receive referral summaries from the Department of Mental Health about a new patient. Diagnoses were page one and became the ground on which clinical hypotheses occur. "Simon has a history of bipolar disorder." With this frame, the goal of my interview is to determine whether Simon's desire to pursue graduate education is a manifestation of his bipolar grandiosity. The clinician risks perceiving everything about Simon in terms of the narrow and unchanging lens of original diagnosis.

Diagnostic reification can also be used by patients to harm themselves. I do not necessarily believe diagnostic labels—calling years of recurring dysphoria, poor appetite, sleep difficulties, diminished self-worth, thoughts of suicide, and major depression—are harmful in themselves. Many people feel significant relief when ongoing and seemingly unexplained behavioral challenges are understood as a potentially meaningful diagnosis. Problems occur, however, when patients listen to the diagnosis and not their own sense of priorities. "I want to get a job working in a downtown business. Wait: someone like me with a diagnosed anxiety disorder cannot handle a job like this." I do not propose throwing out the diagnostic label, only that people who use labels are mindful of possible reified dangers.

INSIGHT INTO SYMPTOMS

One might think that psychiatric symptoms and related dysfunctions dominate a person's life and are prominent on their mind. However, many people with psychiatric diagnoses are unaware that specific experiences are symptomatic of mental illness; they lack insight into their illness. Although hearing voices or having strange beliefs are obviously abnormal to one's friends and family, the patient fails to recognize this as symptomatic of some broader confluence of problems described by psychiatric diagnoses. Researchers and clinicians have described poor insight into a diagnostic condition, anosognosia, the neurological impairment that prevents people from objectively understanding their psychiatric illness.

With insight, one might think comes acceptance, admitting to one's self that current challenges might result from a specific disorder like schizophrenia. Only then can the person recognize the depth and breadth of its impact. Some providers believe people must accept the disease before it can be adequately treated (Gottschaldt, 1997). At a minimum, this requires patients to recognize the syndrome and its disabling effects—to admit to their diagnosis. People lacking insight are not able to do that.

The pursuit of acceptance, however, may lead to unnecessary struggles between service providers and patients. Some people do not want to admit to the label. Perhaps it is an attempt to hold on to one's sense of personal empowerment or perhaps they wish to avoid the loss of personal worth that comes with the label. Perhaps it is a legitimate disagreement about diagnosis and its implications. Whatever the reason, focus on disease acceptance can detour into unnecessary struggles from providers who believe progress only occurs when the patient admits that it undermines the essential partnership necessary for patient and provider to work together. Patients may report feeling unheard by their doctors, and often discontinue treatment as a result.

COURSE OF THE PSYCHIATRIC DISORDER

Diagnoses and the disorders they represent are not static but change over the course of a person's life, depending on internal and external

I Don't Have No Mental Illness

I have a doctorate in clinical psychology and have completed significant course work and training on psychopathology, diagnosis, and testing. I was a postdoc at an esteemed schizophrenia research program at UCLA. I was published in first-rank psychiatry journals. I sure knew what serious and disabling mental illness was. And yet, I did not realize I had a mental illness until twenty years after first seeking help for it! Sure. I knew something was going on; I remember a benevolent priest once taking me to see a psychiatrist while I was a first-year med student. The doc prescribed me Valium; I knew what that was for. But I never saw myself as having mental illness.

That changed when I met a second-year psychiatry resident at an emergency care clinic where I was seeking help. I remember thinking we were mismatched—she seemed like a rookie, not capable of being my doctor—and I was going to teach her something. After thirty minutes she said, "Well, Patrick, it seems like your major depression is back."

"No, not me. I'm not depressed." . . .

It was like a call from heaven, a thunderclap, when I first realized she was right, that I have one of those things that I am expert to heal. Some patients talk about relief when they can finally put a name to the symptoms that challenge them, and that was the case for me.

So why did it take so long for me to have insight? Clearly, it was not because I knew little about mental illness or that I could not understand my emotional state. I also do not think lack of insight occurred because I did not want to admit my mental health failings to boost my self-image. It does seem to be anosognosia—that the observing ego of my brain was not capable of understanding what was going on. I am not sure whether it represented some flaw in my frontal lobes. My depression and anxiety were right in front of me, and I did not see it.

> Let me be clear. Although some version of anosognosia makes sense for me, I do NOT believe it is explanatory for all patient experiences of illness awareness. And I do not want to set up my experience with poor insight as a justification for questioning someone else's journey about understanding their experiences.

circumstances. The disease course is described in terms of *onset* of the disorder, the ongoing *trajectory* once illness has begun, and *end state*. These concepts offer a picture of behavioral health challenges grounded in time and are an important element to understanding the person's experience. However, considerations of course can also cause us to misunderstand the person's experience and lead to stigma.

DISEASE ONSET

The period preceding onset of a full-blown psychiatric disease is known as the *prodrome* during which more subtle manifestations of the symptoms may appear. The prodromal course may be brief and acute or chronic and insidious. It can last for a few months or extend over several years. The disease impact tends to be more of a shock to people with acute onsets, in which psychiatric symptoms seemingly come out of nowhere. Typically, these people experience few psychiatric problems prior to the full-blown set of symptoms characteristic of the illness. The subsequent trajectory of a person with acute onset is frequently more benign than that of the person with chronic onset.

ONGOING TRAJECTORY

Although some serious mental illnesses are short in duration, most last for years, assuming a chronic course. In fact, chronicity is often a defining characteristic of serious mental illness because the dysfunction remains troubling for a significant period of time in the person's life. Trajectory typically follows one of two patterns. Some people experience a relatively simple or flat trajectory where symptoms, dysfunctions, and disabilities do not change much from the onset. Others experience an undulating pattern where they wax and wane. Undulating patterns can be regular and episodic, i.e., described by regular shifts from disease states to remission. Possible factors that might explain this pattern include biological patterns (e.g., monthly hormonal changes) or social schedules (e.g., regular stresses at work, or anniversaries of earlier traumatic events) (Mueser, Rosenberg, Goodman, & Trumbetta, 2002). Irregular patterns are more common.

Decrements of symptoms and dysfunctions from severe levels are described by two phases. During the *residual phase*, symptoms and dysfunctions have markedly decreased from the acute level, but the person still experiences problems that result from the disorder. The person has fewer psychiatric problems than in the acute phase of the illness but is still likely to be disabled by the disorder. Other people with serious mental illness experience total *remission* of symptoms and dysfunctions during benign periods of their course; namely, the person has returned to preprodromal levels. Generally, evidence of remission during the trajectory suggests a better end state than when only residual phases are experienced.

END STATE

What becomes of people with serious mental illnesses? Early psychiatric models mostly suggested negative results. Schizophrenia, for example, was thought to result in a progressive downhill course. Emil Kraepelin (1896) called schizophrenia *dementia praecox* or a precocious dementia because he believed, like most dementing illnesses, that the loss of dysfunction was irretrievable. Several long-term research projects tested this assertion on schizophrenia (Calabrese & Corrigan, 2005). People with schizophrenia were typically identified while in a psychiatric hospital and then followed from ten to thirty years later to determine end state. If Kraepelin were correct, we would expect the vast majority of people with schizophrenia to still be symptomatic, dysfunctional, and not working or living independently at follow-up. Instead, a rough rule of thirds emerged. About one-third of people diagnosed with the most serious psychiatric disorders seem to recover from the disorder in ways similar to patients with serious respiratory disorder; they require short-term aggressive care until the disorder remits. A second third needed to carefully monitor the disorder under the watchful partnership of a health care team, similar to the person challenged by type 2 diabetes. Interventions include some mix of strategic pharmacology and behavioral interventions that promote a healthy lifestyle. The last third are those with "serious" mental illness. Most still recover with the kind of state-of-the-art rehabilitation strategies that have been carefully tested in the literature. It is the bottom third of this last third—about 11 percent—who show the Kraepelinian pattern of progressive downhill course.

Prognosis is the science of predicting a patient's subsequent functioning based on current diagnosis and presentation of symptoms. I urge caution in prognoses especially in terms of clinical practice. Clinicians use prognostications to inform colleagues, patients, and family members about a patient's future prospects. With this information, individuals with serious mental illness are often dissuaded from pursuing personal goals because they may exceed the perceived limitations caused by the illness. A person with schizophrenia cannot get through college or work a full-time job. Attempting goals beyond expected capabilities might lead to failure and relapse. Lay people further exacerbate this by making judgments that rob others of their rightful opportunities. Consider a graduate student of mine with near-perfect transcripts and a growing list of journal publications. She was a person with schizophrenia who was told by a clinical psychology professor that "someone like you could never get through a PhD program" and that "you should save yourself the bother of what inevitably will be failed educational pursuit." I am pleased to say she proved him wrong having earned her doctoral hood and successfully completing a Stanford postdoc.

The problem of prognosis extends to theories of public violence, an especially virulent phenomena after heinous crimes such as mass shootings. Pundits take to airwaves after these tragedies asserting that these kinds of violent acts are to be expected of people with mental illness and require planned interdiction. Prognosis in these various forms deprives people of hope, which is one of the more pernicious legacies of psychiatry—the demoralization that comes with diagnoses. Prognosis in this light leads to institution-bound treatments "to keep the person safe" rather than to community-based strategies in which the person could pursue their own goals. Such prognoses encourage discriminatory actions by employers, who avoid hiring people with mental illness because they fear that these new hires will do bad work. Prognoses are incorporated into public policy to identify and intervene against mentally ill individuals, whom they see as potentially homicidal, in ways that will lead to egregious violations of civil liberties. We must be wary of the pernicious effects of prognosis, both in our practice and in the public's use of seemingly science-based ideas to promulgate stigmatizing and discriminatory statements.

WHAT IS RECOVERY?

Recovery is a movement that displaced the negative prognoses of past psychiatry. It mostly originated from people with lived experience who were frustrated with the gloom and doom of mental health providers, literally stealing peoples' futures. Fortunately, long-term follow-up research substantiated the recovery movement lending a professional imprimatur to this grassroots vision. In this light, recovery seems to be an observable and measurable end state. Bob Liberman (2008), for example, identified criteria that defined recovery from schizophrenia: remission of positive and negative symptoms, working in normative employment settings, and independent living without supervision. Liberman, by the way, was my mentor when I was at UCLA. Bob believed these criteria were achievable, should define the bar for all people with serious mental illness, and therefore are the driving goals for comprehensive pharmacological and rehabilitation programs.

Research, however, seems to challenge such black-and-white end states. Studies, for example, have been unable to show correlations between recovered ends and measures of symptom levels, cognitive dysfunction, or psychosocial skills that comprise Liberman's criteria (Harding et al., 1987a, 1987b). Absence of symptoms is also a problematic recovery criterion because many people with schizophrenia have learned ways to cope with and manage symptoms when they arise and maintain a steady life. The *International Study of Schizophrenia* (Harrison et al., 2001), for example, found that 20 percent of subjects maintained work goals despite persisting symptoms and/or disability.

In this light, a parallel definition of recovery as process emerged (Davidson, 2003). Recovery is a lived experience that evolves over time driven by hope, empowerment, and achievement. Recovery reintroduces optimism into the narrative. People diagnosed with serious mental illnesses such as schizophrenia should not abandon future-sightedness even if significant symptoms and disabilities recur. Consider people with paraplegia who are challenged by repeated dysfunctions. Advocates would cry foul if pessimistic views emerged that suggested people in wheelchairs cannot succeed. Christopher Reeve, Superman from the 1980s films who became quadriplegic after a 1995 equestrian accident, had unending conviction in his future despite disabilities that occurred from losing control of both arms and legs ("Christopher Reeve, thrown from a horse, is suffering paralysis," 1995).

There is an additional concern of recovery as a definable end state that can be measured by a set of criteria. Does recovery mean college degree and full-time job? The world is replete with many people who have not completed college regardless of mental illness and who do not see diplomas as emblematic of what a successful life means for them. There are no achievements that suggest a person is recovered: not education or work or independent living or marriage. Instead, recovery as a process asserts that everyone is capable of pursuing personally meaningful goals. Recovery changed the quality of dialogue between people and their providers from focusing on the can'ts to achieving the cans. Negative prognoses put blinders on health care providers by focusing their attention on what their patients can't do. Patients with schizophrenia can't work, can't live independently, can't get married, or have a family, or get through school, or be successful. Providers became the bastion of safe life decisions, of keeping the person from harm. Caution and warnings were the currency of treatment. Recovery changed this discussion. By reintroducing hope and achievement, providers joined with their patients to talk about what is possible, about what can be done. And with this reframe, treatment became a partnership focused on questions like how do we help you get a job, live independently, find intimate relationships, and enjoy good health?

HOW MIGHT WE HELP PEOPLE WITH SERIOUS MENTAL ILLNESS?

Research over the last fifty years has led to many strategies that may help people with serious mental illness to accomplish their personal goals. In this light, mental health professions have called for *evidence-based practices* (EBPs) to define interventions that are, in fact, effective. Why is the search for EBPs important? The history of mental health treatment is filled with quackery, including but not limited to animal magnetism, bloodletting, trephining (drilling through the skull), hydrotherapy (dunking patients in extremely cold water), and insulin shock therapy. Ineffective treatments remain to this day including dialysis, vitamin therapy, and therapeutic crystals. There are also interventions that, while not patently egregious, do not show significant benefits for serious mental illness. Freudian psychoanalysis is one.

A multiyear Substance Abuse and Mental Health Services–funded effort attempted to catalog EBPs for the serious mental illnesses (Drake et al., 2001). The EBPs that made the list can roughly be differentiated into two categories: psychosocial interventions and psychotropic medications. There are excellent textbooks that describe specific strategies within these two domains. Here, I briefly summarize the two, beginning with psychosocial interventions, the array of "talk" therapies that help people achieve goals blocked by mental illness. I then review medical interventions that are often sources of concern and suspicion by some people with lived conditions. Current practice related to electroconvulsive therapy (ECT) and psychosurgery are especially provocative examples related to stigma and included here.

PSYCHOSOCIAL INTERVENTIONS

There are fundamental provider skills that are the basis of psychosocial services for people with serious mental illness. Typically such interventions begin with *goal setting*, practical activities providers use to help people identify and act on personal aspirations. Goal assessment assures that the focus of treatment is driven by the client's perceptions of important needs. Essential to the pursuit of goals is *support* offered formally by mental health providers, or less so by family, friends, and peers. Instrumental support is the practical aid that helps people directly meet goals: rides to a job interview, help with visiting a new dentist, or getting through weekly laundry chores. Interpersonal support is the nonspecific quality of relationships necessary for the pursuit of goals in one's community, warm and genuine relationships with others that lead to feelings of worth and belonging.

Skills training helps adults who lack social and coping skills to learn adaptive behaviors so they can increase their support network and deal more effectively with life's demands. Skills training is based on social learning theory and comprises several steps. Actors model skills so that participants can witness them. Participants are then encouraged to rehearse the newly learned skills during role plays; for example, participants learning basic conversation skills may be instructed to role-play a conversation about local sports teams with an acquaintance on a bus. Social and material rewards are subsequently distributed for successful participation in the role play.

Persons with severe mental illnesses are often hampered by cognitive deficits including problems with attention, memory, decision making, and expression. Social and coping skills may not be fully learned because participants have difficulty recognizing similarities and differences between the training setting and other important situations. *Cognitive rehabilitation and therapy* helps participants resolve the information processing deficits that hamper the performance of important skills. Researchers have attempted to improve participants' deficits in attention, memory, and conceptual flexibility. *Mindfulness* has been incorporated into cognitive therapy to enhance its effects. Although largely emerging from Buddhist philosophies, mindfulness has been adapted for Western therapies (Kabat-Zinn, 2013). Mindfulness is the intentional, accepting and nonjudgmental focus of a person's attention on the emotions, thoughts, and sensations occurring in the present moment.

Pursuing goals and overcoming symptoms and disabilities is difficult; people often relapse. *Relapse prevention* (RP) is a cognitive-behavioral intervention in which rehabilitation providers help people plan for and control relapses during periods where they are relatively strong. RP was originally developed to help people attempting to control alcohol and drug use (Larimer, Palmer, & Marlatt, 1999). It has since also been applied to mental health issues. In this case, relapse might be experienced as being overwhelmed again by anxiety, depression, or voices. RP helps people define slips, identify high-risk situations where slips might occur, plan ways to avoid these high-risk situations, and practice coping skills when relapses occur.

Providers weave fundamental skills into programs meant to help people with serious mental illness achieve "big picture" goals—those related to education, vocation, relationships, independent living, health, wellness, and other goals that sum to yield a quality life. They translate into support programs, e.g., supported housing, supported employment, and supported education. An additionally important set of interventions focuses on the interacting needs of people with serious mental illness and their families. They might include psychoeducation programs, which teach families and patients ways to manage day-to-day problems, or interfamily support, in which families learn from person-to-person exchanges with other families.

PSYCHIATRIC MEDICATIONS

Psychiatrists and other medical practitioners have a vast array of medications that might be used to help patients manage symptoms including antipsychotics, antidepressants, mood stabilizers, anxiolytics (antianxiety medications), and psychostimulants. I will discuss each briefly in turn. Antipsychotic medications are often prescribed for disorders in the schizophrenia spectrum and for people showing psychotic symptoms because of depression or bipolar disorder. They seem to have the best effects on symptoms such as delusions, hallucinations, and formal thought disorder. There are two major subgroups to the antipsychotics: conventional and atypical. The latter are called second generation because they emerged after conventional medications, out of a line of research that gained prominence in the late 1980s. Atypical medications seem to cause less-harmful side effects than conventional drugs, and they offer some benefits on the negative symptoms of schizophrenia like flat affect, limited speech, and few interactions.

There are three subgroups of antidepressant medications. The oldest are monoamine oxidase inhibitors (MAOIs); they have dangerous side effects and, hence, are used sparingly. The second subgroup, tricyclic and tetracyclic medications, have relatively similar chemistry and physiological effects that differ from the third subgroup, selective serotonin reuptake inhibitors (SSRIs). Antidepressant medications are often indicated for people showing marked biological (e.g., sleep disturbances), psychological (sadness and hopelessness), and behavioral symptoms (suicide). This may include people with major depression or anxiety disorders.

Lithium carbonate is often the first mood stabilizer prescribed for the manic symptoms of bipolar disorder and related illnesses. It seems to diminish the expansive mood and troubling behaviors that occur to people in a manic state. Other mood stabilizers with less-harmful effects, such as Tegretol and Depakote, have since emerged.

Benzodiazepines are a group of medications that once were used to help people manage their anxiety but are less often prescribed now because they can be addictive. There are nonbenzodiazepines like BuSpar that seem to be less addicting. Sometimes benzodiazepines and nonbenzodiazepines are prescribed to help people fall asleep. However, they are prescribed sparingly because they may worsen sleep when taken for a long time.

Psychostimulants are medications that reduce fatigue, promote alertness, and enhance mood. They have been used narrowly to assist people with attention deficit hyperactivity disorder (ADHD) or narcolepsy. People taking psychostimulants for ADHD show less impulsivity and better attentiveness. Narcolepsy is a chronic sleep disorder marked by overwhelming daytime drowsiness and sudden sleep attacks. Psychostimulants may decrease sleepiness in this group.

SIDE EFFECTS

Psychiatric medications may negatively affect every organ system in the body. Antipsychotic medications can make people feel tired and fatigued, lower blood pressure, and lead to skin rashes. They also have neurological effects including muscles spasms, tremors, and restlessness. Atypical antipsychotics can lead to sedation, changes in appetite, constipation, and obesity (in worst cases leading to type 2 diabetes). MAOIs for depression have significant side effects including blood pressure crises that are worsened by some foods and medications. Tricyclics also impact blood pressure, though at less-risky levels. Tricyclics may have neurological side effects including tremor or sedation. They may also cause weight gain, esophageal reflux, and sexual dysfunctions. SSRIs have in some ways become more popular because they seem to have fewer side effects than the other two subgroups. That said, they still may have negative effects on digestion, sleep, restlessness, and sexual functioning.

Lithium has risky cardiac effects that typically require regular blood tests. In addition, lithium and the other mood stabilizers might negatively affect digestive, dermatological, and neurological systems. Anxiolytics also suppress respiration. Nonbenzodiazepines have risks of their own including, paradoxically, nervousness and insomnia. Psychostimulants need to be used cautiously in people with psychosis because they can worsen symptoms such as hallucinations. Psychostimulants, in general, can also have heart, digestive, and neurological effects.

Side effects are not trivial. Their consideration in competent medication management has changed dramatically over the course of my professional life. When I was a student, I saw patients who were on numbing levels of medication in the belief that dosages should be increased until symptoms disappeared. "Side effects be damned; getting rid of the psychosis was primary." Medical providers are now more sensitive and sympathetic to the discomfort and disability caused by side effects. Instead of being told, "You'll need to be on antidepressants for the rest of your life," patients are now fully educated about medication options and schedules. Perhaps a patient will take an antipsychotic medication for six months, for example, and deal with the relatively minor side effects along the way, instead of taking the medication unendingly.

MEDICAL DEVICES

There are two "medical devices" for serious mental illness that are frequently the center of public concern about rights and stigma: ECT and psychosurgery. Although both have a controversial past, some evidence suggests that they may be effective—albeit in much more controlled formats than they were previously administered. Previously known as electroshock therapy, ECT induces seizures in patients by electrically stimulating the brain through one or two electrodes placed on the head. The procedure is conducted in a well-controlled environment, with the patient given sedatives prior to stimulus to avoid self-harm. ECT has a prominent history of misuse in psychiatry; it was infamously depicted in Ken Kesey's book *One Flew over the Cuckoo's Nest*, in which ECT was used to cow a raucous patient, Randall McMurphy, under the vigilant eye of ward nurse Ratched.

At one time ECT was indiscriminately used on psychiatric patients with almost every conceivable diagnosis, in many cases more to control the obstreperous patient than to address symptoms. In a resulting backlash, ECT experienced a period of relative disuse. However, research in the past twenty years has shown that judicious use of ECT may have beneficial effects for people with major depression, especially those whose symptoms do not remit after state-of-the-art pharmaco- or psychotherapy (Waite & Easton, 2013). These are people literally paralyzed by dysphoria and vegetative symptoms that prevent them from accomplishing even basic living skills.

Lobotomy was one form of psychosurgery, in which the skull was surgically opened and connections to anterior lobes of the brain were severed. In orbital lobotomies, a particularly gruesome example of the procedure, the patient's head was immobilized and pick-like probes were hammered through bony plates behind the eye to destroy anterior lobes of the brain. Lobotomies were hailed by the medical profession when the procedure was first introduced; Antonio Egas Moniz won the 1949 Nobel Prize in Physiology or Medicine for his work on a form of lobotomy. Like ECT, lobotomy has been flayed in the media. *Cuckoo's Nest* ends with Randall McMurphy in a permanently vegetative state because of a frontal lobotomy, and the lobotomy is featured in the more recent film *Shutter Island* with Leonardo DiCaprio. Lobotomy has claimed famous victims including Eva Peron, 1930s film actress Frances Farmer, and Rosemary Kennedy, sister of President John Kennedy. Like ECT, lobotomies all but disappeared from psychiatric settings for forty years.

Psychosurgery has reemerged as a possible strategy for intransigent psychiatric problems such as disabling obsessive compulsive disorder. Rather than its coarse and barbaric predecessor, however, modern psychosurgery is now conducted much more precisely. In limbic leucotomy, for example, three 6-mm lesions are made in the lower medial quadrant of the frontal lobe. Instead of brutal hammer-driven probes, lesions are made using temperature-controlled probes. Physicians seem to agree that psychosurgery is best indicated for the patient with aggression that is unresponsive to other interventions.

Although many people have rightfully decried the savagery of ECT and psychosurgery as they were formerly performed, treatments should not be discarded if they can be potentially helpful. ECT and psychosurgery may serve this purpose in limited situations. Neither should any treatment be forced on patients. Patients should be the final arbiters of their own treatment plans. ECT and lobotomies were performed on helpless patients strapped down to tables, helplessly victimized by these invasive treatments. Contemporary practice, in contrast, prioritizes self-determination and person-centered care.

REVISITING THE EVIDENCE BASE

What better criteria can there be for selecting treatments than showing the evidence? The bar, however, is more difficult to reach than one might think. Consider research on the impact of psychiatric medication. The design is relatively straightforward involving random assignment of participants to ingest either the index medication (e.g., an antipsychotic or antidepressant) or comparison medication(s). Effects of these medications on symptoms and disabilities are assessed at baseline and subsequent follow-ups (e.g., one and six months after beginning the medication). Researchers also assess patterns of adverse events after beginning a medication; does ingesting the medication lead to annoying or harmful side effects? Meeting the evidence bar is fairly clear. Positive evidence: the medication leads to significant reduction in symptoms and disabilities. Negative evidence: the medication causes adverse events.

The medication research industry is so large that the National Institute of Mental Health has convened Patient Outcomes Research Teams for more than fifteen years to sift through the literature and generate consensus guidelines on using medications as well as other psychosocial treatments. Robert Buchanan led a team of scientists reviewing more than 600 studies on antipsychotic medication for schizophrenia completed between 1998 and 2010 (Buchanan et al., 2010). Their recommendations included prescription patterns for acute psychotic symptoms, protocols for first-episode schizophrenia, and maintenance strategies for people with schizophrenia who are responsive to medications.

However, perhaps all is not so serene. Investigative reporter Robert Whitaker wrote a biting review of research on antipsychotic medication in 2002. He noted that the preponderance of studies on psychiatric medication is completed by the pharmaceutical industry, companies that are motivated to find good evidence in order to increase sales and enhance profit. Whitaker focused on studies meant to test the effects of conventional and atypical antipsychotic medication. Atypicals were believed to have better impact on symptoms with fewer side effects. They were also newer products. Depending on the medication, atypicals were two to five times more expensive than conventional medications (Brown, Markowitz, Moore, & Parker, 1999). Hence, there was significant financial benefit for pharmaceutical companies to find the evidence for atypical antipsychotic medications.

Studies with randomized assignment were completed by Janssen, Eli Lilly, and AstraZeneca on their atypicals. They used this evidence to conclude that atypical antipsychotic medication has superior impact on symptoms with fewer side effects than the conventional medicine, haloperidol. Food and Drug Administration (FDA) interpretations, however, were far less sanguine. About Janssen research on its atypical, Risperdal, Robert Temple, director of the FDA Office of Drug Evaluation said,

> We would consider any advertisement or promotion labeling for Risperdal false, misleading, or lacking fair balance . . . if there is presentation of data that conveys the impression that risperidone is superior to haloperidol or any other marketed antipsychotic drug product with regard to safety or effectiveness.
>
> (Whitaker, 2002)

The FDA seemed equally harsh in its review of AstraZeneca's research on quetiapine. They ruled that four of eight studies failed to provide meaningful evidence relevant to quetiapine's effect. The remaining four studies were unable to show superior effects for atypical compared to conventional antipsychotics. In addition, side effects were equally bad for both groups.

In order to overcome concerns about pharmaceutical company research, the National Institute of Mental Health funded the only large-scale randomized study contrasting the effects of atypical and conventional medication on symptoms and side effects; it was the Clinical Antipsychotic Trials Intervention Effectiveness (CATIE) study (Lieberman & Stroup, 2011). CATIE enrolled more than 1600 research participants in the study. Findings were not positive. About 75 percent of people given atypical antipsychotic medication decided to quit the medication before the end of the study because of adverse side effects. Think of this: how would consumers respond to any product—cleaning aid, sports equipment, automobile, medication—where three of four test subjects rejected it, not because it did not work very well but because the product was noxious? Of those who did complete the study, no difference was found in symptom or disability change comparing people receiving atypical versus conventional antipsychotic medication. Despite murky evidence at best, "research findings" still changed the course of prescription patterns. Prescriptions for conventional antipsychotic medication almost halved between 1995 and 2001 while atypicals almost tripled (Grohmann, Engel, Geissler, & Ruther, 2004).

Although atypicals were touted because they reduced side effects compared to conventional antipsychotics, CATIE findings were again sobering (Nasrallah, 2009). Atypicals do not show the harmful movement disorders of conventional medications. However, they have significant effects on appetite often leading to what is known as the metabolic syndrome, a collection of symptoms that correspond to obesity including large waistline, increased triglycerides (fat found in blood), high blood pressure, and high fasting blood sugar. People with metabolic syndrome are at much higher risk for type 2 diabetes mellitus, coronary heart disease, and stroke. CATIE data showed research participants receiving the atypical antipsychotic Olanzapine had a 10 percent increase in metabolic syndrome. Hence, while atypicals may not cause harmful movement disorders, they may lead to systemic illnesses leading to significant morbidity and even death.

New York psychiatrist Peter Breggin and his wife Ginger Ross Breggin (1994) wrote a similarly stinging review of research on antidepressant medication, once again indicting pharmaceutical companies in manipulating evidence to suit market goals. They summarized the FDA's 1988 review of fourteen studies submitted by Eli Lilly as evidence that supports Prozac; its antidepressant effects are due to selective serotonin reuptake inhibition. SSRIs are in some ways like atypical antipsychotic medications representing a second generation of antidepressants believed to be more effective and less aversive than traditional tricyclic antipsychotic medication like Tofranil. SSRIs also represented market growth potential. The FDA concluded that only three of these studies showed support for Prozac. Six of seven studies demonstrated Prozac to be less effective than Tofranil. Side effects were sobering. Despite statements about fewer harmful effects, Prozac may cause headache, nervousness, insomnia, nausea, diarrhea, and sexual dysfunction. Some patients might decide these effects are minor and worth withstanding in order to enjoy antidepressant results. However, Prozac also

I am personally not ready to omit medications from my health plan. I got up this morning and took my 20-mg dose of Prozac and 200 mgs of Lamotrigine prescribed by Dr. McSay. Nor am I ready to discourage my patients from considering benefits and costs of anti-psychotic or antidepressant medications in their lives. There is, after all, impressive work by PORT and others that shows some evidence supporting medication. I add to this, anecdotal comments from colleagues and my own experiences, which have concluded that benefits of medications outweigh costs for me and for some other people.

This decision, however, does not reflect the cool examination of evidence. It is also based on lore. I am steeped in a medical world that says drugs are what's needed when overwhelmed by symptoms. I am desperate for myself and my patients not to be overwhelmed by the stress and disabilities of serious mental illness. Lore leads to super-stition. If I stop taking the meds, it will all come back.

However, after reading Whitaker and Breggin, I am more con-vinced that I (and my patients) need to be captain of the treatment plan. We are the people who solely benefit from the plan as well as are harmed by unintended effects.

seems to lead to greater increase in suicide. In fact, in 2004 the FDA issued a "black box" warning about SSRIs in general, especially for children and young adults. Namely, patients taking SSRIs are at greater risk for suicide.

These findings echo what philosophers and historians of science have been saying for the past fifty years (Kuhn, 1962). Science is not an innocent pursuit. It occurs in the same set of political and commercial forces as most social enterprises. Choice of topic, specification of design, and interpreta-tion of results cannot escape zeitgeist. Consider this from another perspective—the authoritarian power of science. Once, people believed something because an authority said so: a god, the king, or wise men. They frequently represented patent observation. "Anyone can see the earth is flat or the sun goes around the earth." Science became important when it proved that method trumps authority. Just because the Vatican said the universe was earth centered did not make it so. Astronomers have proven the obverse.

Ironically, science has become an authoritarian enterprise because of its complexity. It seems that research methods and statistics are so complicated that the average person is unable to decipher its significance. Hence, the average person relies on the authority of the science. There is a sanguine reliance when scientists agree. However, people are misled when there is discord in the data.

What does this all mean for evidence? The reader must be more alert to the positive and negative effects of medication. By the way, similar concerns need to guide personal decisions about psychosocial treatments. Hence, people with serious mental illness need to be active consumers of research, sifting through differing perspectives on what evidence means. But not everyone has the time or skills to do this for themselves. Hence, they should seek out consumer reports from differing sources to gain a broader perspective of interventions.

TREATMENT ADHERENCE

Given the evidence, it should not be a surprise that many people may decide not to seek out treatment despite the research (Institute of Medicine, 2007). Findings from major nationwide studies—the Epidemiologic Catchment Area Study (Narrow, Regier, Rae, Manderscheid, & Locke, 1993), the National Comorbidity Survey (Kessler et al., 2001), and the National Comorbidity Survey Replication (Kessler & Merikangas, 2004)—show that 30 to 40 percent of people who, for example, might benefit from psychotropic medication, fail to see a doctor for it. Advocacy groups from many organizations—including the American Psychological Association, Mental Health America, and the National Alliance on Mental Illness—have made this issue a priority. The National Institutes of Health agreed and launched its Adherence Research Network (ARN) in 2007 to investigate adherence for all kinds of health conditions (National Institutes of Health, 2010). The ARN's charge is clear; if people participate in treatment as prescribed, then treatment's impact on health would grow exponentially. If people with mental illness just took their medication, the egregious impact of psychiatric disorders could be controlled.

The concept of *adherence* has a long and tortuous history in psychiatric services. It was once believed that people who did not participate in services were *resisting* care and risking symptom remission and relapse. Personality weaknesses were hypothesized to block the person from fully engaging in treatment, mostly "ego protective" factors that developed from early interactions with one's mother. Some theorists tried to transcend accusatory notions of resistance and instead put forth the concept of compliance. *Compliance* was meant more as an objective indicator, a categorical assessment—yes or no—of whether the person has taken medications or otherwise participated in treatment as prescribed. Remitting symptoms was still the fundamental concern as well as the fear that treatment failure could lead to an irreversible tragedy like suicide. For some, compliance meant urging patients to do their treatment, by hook or by crook, regardless of its impact on self-determination. Compliance thus could easily be confused with coercion. Strategies meant to serve compliance included inpatient and outpatient commitment, more benign coercion (e.g., exercise of a guardian's authority), diminished personal control (e.g., monthly injections of antipsychotic medication), or benevolent trickery (e.g., not sharing the full range of side effects).

The concept of adherence emerged as clinicians noted that patients wanted to actively participate in their treatment decisions. Service providers might still dominate in the development of treatment goals, but they should seek to involve patients when possible. Despite its promise, adherence is still a problematic idea. It suggests that the patient who does not take prescribed medication or participate in a rehabilitation program is doing something wrong. "John is making a stupid choice by not taking his antipsychotic medication for schizophrenia." Disapproval of treatment choices can lead to disrespect of the person.

Collaboration evolved organically from adherence by recognizing that expertise is shared by provider and patient. Psychiatrists are experts in symptoms, biological processes, and possibly healing; patients best know their own illness, their lives, and how previous treatments have worked. The idea of collaboration was an insightful perspective for its time, elevating patients to equal status with their providers and, through this peer relationship, generating effective plans.

Collaboration segued to *engagement*, the gold standard in current discussions about health beliefs and decisions. The gradual move from compliance and adherence to engagement reflects a primary shift in focus from outcome to process. Compliance considered outcome to be the essential value; namely, did treatment lead to improved symptoms? Engagement recognizes that the process—the nature of the ongoing interaction between provider and patient—is equally important. This discussion moved from whether patients are doing what they *should* to what are the processes that affect independent decision making and behaviors related to health. Instead of wondering how we might convince a patient to take a particular treatment, we consider how we can help people determine for themselves the best plan of action.

Self-determination is choice! This is stated as an ethical manifesto—that by the very essence of being human, people have the right to choose where they want to live, what they want to do, with whom they wish to affiliate, and how they wish to enjoy spiritual, educational, and recreational pursuits. These are first-order principles laid out in the constitutions of most governments, the United Nations Charter, and President George W. Bush's 2003 New Freedom Commission meant to chart the course of mental health services. People with serious mental illnesses must have choice over personal goals and traditional or nontraditional approaches to facilitate these goals. But choice is not just an ethic; it is psychological reality. People will retreat from social exchanges where specific behaviors are forced on them. This is known as psychological reactance. People are choosing all the time; they vote with their feet. They drop out of school if it does not meet their vocational goals. They exercise daily if it is consistent with their idea of wellness. They take medication when it seems to have a positive impact. Understanding this reality is where social scientists are needed, modeling the choice process in terms of deciding and acting on health issues.

Shared decision making (SDM) is an evidence-based practice that is essential for promoting self-determination and is comprised of three steps: (1) Assist decision making by helping the person examine costs and benefits of health options. The person is encouraged to identify and make sense of the advantages and disadvantages of a specific service for specific problems caused by the illness. (2) This assessment is facilitated by information so the person better understands disease, corresponding treatment, and other relevant parameters. (3) Health-related decision making is, fundamentally, social intercourse between person and provider. Skills that enhance qualities of the exchange may positively affect treatment decision. Shared decision making is revolutionary in practice, especially for clinicians from the old school. It means psychiatrists need to be prepared for and respect patient decisions that sometimes may differ from clinical wisdom. It means psychiatrists need to accept and support the person who decides to stop taking antipsychotic medication, even if ceasing medication last time led to a recurrence of hallucinations and delusions pushing the person back into the hospital.

DIGNITY TO FAIL

Despite the value of shared decision making, many service providers remain concerned that decisions that lead to the "wrong" treatment result in unnecessary symptoms and disabilities. This could lead to suicide, homicide, or other equally tragic consequences and therefore is not to be taken lightly. Mental health advocates are troubled, however, that this concern leads to overprotective decisions. Consider how physical disability advocates consider the issue when they discuss dignity of risk and right to failure (Townsend, 2010). Attempting to make life "risk free" robs people of potential opportunities. People do not land a better job, move to a nicer neighborhood, build more intimate relationships, or enjoy fewer medication side effects if they do not entertain and pursue risky options. Many a person's best achievements come the hard way—falling flat, picking one's self up, and moving on. Without these flops, people are unclear about limits to what they might do and miss out on unforeseen and potentially benefiting alternatives.

Might "pursuit of risk" be unreal for people with serious mental illness, especially people who seem to be unable to make clear decisions because of recurring cognitive dysfunctions? This is a complex question. Decision capacity is not a black-and-white process. Even people with major psychoses have lucid periods. And who decides whether a person's decision represents a pathological process? Is a decision to stop medications by a person suffering significant side effects necessarily indicative of poor thought processes? In addition, research shows opting out of a treatment does not necessarily lead to worse symptoms (Corrigan, Angell et al., 2012). In situations where illness intensifies, the person rarely cascades into irreversible calamity. Most decisions about ending psychosocial treatments related to work or independent living do not lead to relapse and catastrophe. Even failure in medication regimens does not necessarily lead to tragedy.

Risk and failure is part of human agency. Saving people from them takes away their dignity. Dignity to fail, however, is not meant as carte blanche for pursuit of goals regardless of its impact on others. Self-determination is bound by the same societal limits that govern all adults. People are expected to make decisions that reflect not only their interest but those of significant others such as friends, family, and coworkers. People need to act responsibly. This expectation equally applies to people with serious mental illness. The idea of responsibility might be viewed as a restraint to self-determination; for individuals with mental health problems this may mean that people are responsible for partaking in treatment so as not to burden others. Yet, taking responsibility for one's own health and well-being is also advocated by the recovery movement (Chamberlin, 1978). Responsibility suggests that people with mental illness are capable of making valuable choices, and therefore deserving of self-determination like everyone else. Self-determination requires a balanced perspective, exercising one's personal agency while responsibly considering the concerns of others.

Some claim that assertions about dignity to fail are naïve. The Treatment Advocacy Center in Arlington Virginia, for example, takes a hard line against mental health systems that have been unable to monitor and control psychiatric patients who have gone on to violently harm others. The founder, distinguished psychiatrist E. Fuller Torrey, is especially fond of citing the pernicious effects of anosognosia. His 2008 book *The Insanity Offense: How America's Failure to Treat the Seriously Mentally Ill Endangers Its Citizens* poignantly makes the case with examples drawn from the news. He relayed a May 2006 account of the funeral of Vicky Armel, a forty-four-year-old police detective shot to death by eighteen-year-old Michael Kennedy, a person with untreated schizophrenia. Armel left behind a loving husband and two young children. Or consider his recollection of the brutal stabbing death of Pamela Ann Jones by her son Nathan, who had mental illness, and was a former student of the College of William and Mary.

Torrey is able to incur a mix of pity and anger in his articulate books. His readers may well question views of empowerment. His insights should not be dismissed lightly. But I also believe the picture he paints is limited and skewed, choosing to portray people with mental illness as something to be feared. In some ways, Torrey's writings are similar to racists who portray low-income black Chicagoans as dangerous by cherry-picking

Don't Ever Quit!

I heard this message throughout much of my schooling and adulthood. Victory goes to those who persevere. Quitters are cowards. Hold out for another day and you will succeed. These are the words that inspired many of my favorite movies. And yet I did. I quit. A lot. And it hurt.

- All my life I wanted to grow up to be a doctor. And I got into medical school. I got overwhelmed, and I quit.
- I then thought I wanted to help people who were mentally ill, so I got into a PhD program in clinical psychology. Overwhelmed again and I quit.
- Went on to be interested in the philosophy of behavioral science, got into a prestigious program at the University of Chicago on an NSF scholarship and quit.
- Got a postdoctoral fellowship at UCLA and quit.

I repeatedly failed because of my mental illness. I am not sure this realization is a relief or a justification. But I would become hugely overwhelmed by the demands of graduate training, doubt my worth and future, wonder if I'd be better off dead, and escape.

To be honest, I would not be able to write of these private shames if I had not somehow gotten to a place where I accomplished something. And this is the heart of recovery—that despite one's challenges, people continue to achieve, though goals that represent achievement might vary. ACHIEVEMENT can be a slippery slope in defining recovery. I recovered because I earned a doctorate and am now a distinguished professor of psychology at a Research 2 doctoral university. This might seem to set the bar high for recovery. But recovery is not a presumptuous master. It does not specify the criteria one must achieve to be considered recovered. Rather, it is a process that recognizes everyone has goals (from Nobel Prize to working daily to attending support programs with peers); pursuit of these goals indicates one is engaged in his or her world—recovered. Recovery is hopeful.

shooting stories of African American assailants published in the summer 2016 issues of the *Tribune*. The whole picture is much more complex than a sampling of shooting tragedies, be they about people with mental illness or African Americans. Both strive for "noble" policy to curtail violence but instead end up stigmatizing groups.

CAN THERE BE FALSE HOPE?

I present hope in this chapter as seemingly limitless potential for promoting well-being. Might not hope have its limits? After all, a diagnosis of schizophrenia, like that of cancer or heart disease, is sobering. Mental health providers and patients are wise to heed lessons that can be learned from these labels. Grief reactions were once thought to be normal responses to diagnoses of serious mental illness, especially on the part of family. Psychiatrists wondered whether working through the fundamental loss experienced through the child with schizophrenia—loss of education, industriousness, relationship—was the healthy way to move on from such tragic news. Hope seems to ring falsely in this perspective.

> My son Jeremy was so full of promise. High school honors, lettered in sports, accepted to an Ivy League school. But now he has schizophrenia. He's done. My soul breaks at this tragedy.

Bioethicist William Ruddick (1999) examined the nuance of false hope. Is it false hope to encourage a patient to enter a medication trial for stage 4 breast cancer by highlighting the possibilities while omitting the negative probabilities? Is it false hope to suggest that a person with formal thought disorder and delusions of reference might go to medical school? Not necessarily. Ruddick said there are advantages to optimism. Hope has clinical benefits; illness seems to wane in the face of optimism. Hope promotes participation in treatment, especially those services that are demanding and protracted. People who more fully participate in treatment receive more attentive care from medical providers.

However, Ruddick said there may be limitations to hope in medicine, especially in cases of deceptive communication about prognosis. Consider the harm wrought by the oncologist withholding prognosis for the woman with stage 4 cancer. Giving her inaccurate information undermines her autonomy. She cannot, for example, be fully informed about clinical and side effects of the cancer medication trial when unaware of the boundaries of her prognosis. Most ethicists agree that autonomy trumps beneficence when assessing costs and benefits of clinical communications. Ruddick tempers these concerns with consideration of the uncertainty of specific medical practices defined by probabilities and possibilities. Probability is the domain of the provider; given hard signs of a disease, what are the chances that specific interventions will yield therapeutic outcomes? Possibility is the arena of patients and their families, often influenced by variables beyond science. How might my health change if I put my faith in treatment or God? Medical providers might accommodate statements about hope and probabilities when met by strong assertions of possibilities from family and patient.

Is hope limited as an idea for people with serious mental illness? In some ways, it seems easier to argue about hope and cancer mortality than hope and psychiatric disabilities. Perhaps it is because issues of death seem a bit clearer than questions about whether a person can go back to work, live independently, or get married. Markers of disease predicting death are a bit more compelling than those of psychiatric symptoms and corresponding disabilities. As stated earlier, psychiatric research has been largely disappointing in identifying predictors of employment and independent living beyond small correlations. As a result, false positives in discouraging a person with schizophrenia from returning to work are high.

False hope has been important when describing limitations of mental and physical health services. Consider, for example, the dismal results of therapeutic efforts to decrease smoking, control alcohol and drug use, manage diet, and promote exercise based on false hope characterized by unrealistic expectations about the ease and consequences of attempts to change. False hope results in continued attempts to pursue avenues of behavior change that are likely to be ineffective for the individual. False hope prevents people from objectively assessing status and goals. Applied to psychiatric disabilities, false hope might suggest people pursue work goals that exceed true abilities. For example, someone seeks a full-time job as a paralegal when a more realistic job may be half-time janitorial assistant. Might they need to replace these erroneous efforts with more realistic goals?

Still, concerns about false hope may be based on incorrect assumptions (Snyder & Rand, 2003). For example, proponents of false hope suggest failed attempts at behavior change are downhill and deleterious. Perhaps frequent and evolving efforts at goal attainment eventually lead to success. False hope models frame behavior variation as black and white, which is contrary to contemporary approaches to change. Abstinence from alcohol, for example, is often tempered with harm-reduction models where people are helped to diminish the impact of alcohol use rather than erase it altogether.

Hope, however, is not blind. It does not mean individuals forego careful self-assessment and critical thinking. Life's decisions are more effective when people have knowledge about the full range of personal challenges and response options. Mental health service providers, peers, and others can help obtain this information. This includes assessment of where the person currently stands in terms of challenges and skills. Others might help the decision maker by providing alternative perspectives of a goal. "You know, Henry, getting an associate's degree to pursue licensed practical nursing might be an intermediate step before attempting to get into medical school." But at the end of the day, the decision lies with Henry.

STRENGTH-BASED INTERVENTIONS

By providing an atmosphere of dignity and hope, the recovery movement impacted intervention principles in terms of assessment and service provision. Replacing can'ts with cans begged for a broader sense of assessment. Measures of symptoms, dysfunctions, and disabilities are ways to understand the limitations, important for the patient seeking mental health service plans to be sure, but are only a part of the picture. Strengths-based assessment is an essential addition to intervention efforts meant to get a complete picture of the person. Strengths are broadly conceived as attributes that might be availed to achieve personally valued goals. *Personal strengths* include determination, punctuality, affability, or good humor. *Social strengths* are support of a family member, interests and enjoyment shared with a friend, loving partners, or concerned clergy. In addition, strengths assessments may reflect the community. *Environmental strengths* include whether a local health club offers discounts for people of low incomes, a pharmacy provides medication daily pillboxes, or a local café has free Internet access. Service providers should not adopt a black-and-white view of strengths. "Yes or no? Harry is determined." Strengths are flexible. For example, to what extent might Harry avail his sense of determination to meet his work goals?

What does a recovery model suggest about who provides the mental health interventions outlined in this chapter? Traditionally, mental health providers were considered to be those with professional credentials and requisite training. Medication management, for example, suggests medical school, residency, and licensing boards. Similar standards exist for clinical psychologists, psychiatric nurses, mental health counselors, and clinical social workers among others. In each case, the practice bar is set by mastery and testing on some body of knowledge.

The recovery movement broadened this list to include peers, services provided by people with lived experience. Who is a peer? They are usually people with past history of significant mental illness that caused psychiatric disability. There are no litmus tests for "peer": hospitalization, medication, length of illness, social security disability, and work disruption. People who self-identify as individuals with lived experience of serious mental illness are considered peers. Peers hired into service positions are also in recovery; they are able to achieve important life goals including those related to employment despite their disabilities.

Peer services are strengths based and combine emotional with instrumental support that is mutually provided by individuals with lived experience who come together to bring about social and personal change. Peer support is mutually beneficial through a reciprocal process of giving and receiving based on principles of respect and shared responsibility. Through this system of sharing, supporting, and assisting others, feelings of rejection, discrimination, frustration, and loneliness are combated. Usually peers providing support in the traditional sense of self-help groups do so as volunteers. Peers who deliver support services are typically financially compensated employees. How might peer support differ from professional services? Peers understand each other because they've "been there," shared similar experiences, and model a willingness to learn and grow. Peers assemble in order to change unhelpful patterns, get out of "stuck" places, and build relationships that are respectful, mutually responsible, and, potentially, mutually transforming.

"When did the nuts take over the nuthouse?" This line from *Batman Begins* captures some of the hostile objections to peer services. People with serious mental illness do not have the knowledge base or skills to meaningfully treat peers. They lack necessary boundaries needed to offer competent intervention. Their own mental illness will cloud the quality of care. These might be reasonable concerns for all provider groups charged with helping people meet their behavioral health challenges. Research on the effectiveness of peer support yields a complex picture of results (Davidson, Bellamy, Guy, & Miller, 2012). Outcomes suggest that peers are able to fill many of the roles that comprise support programs as competently as paraprofessionals doing these jobs without lived experience. Future research will examine whether there are aspects of the peer experience that yield outcomes unable to be realized by nonpeer professionals, e.g., promotion of hope, encouragement of self-determination, and control of stigma. Ongoing study of peer services needs to separate legitimate questions about feasibility and impact from the more insidious concerns of some professional groups about the presumed incompetence of peers to do many mental health interventions.

SOCIAL DISADVANTAGE

So far, I have written about serious mental illness and substance use disorders as a psychologist steeped in behavioral and neurosciences. Sociologists and social work scholars have an additional perspective of psychiatric disorders that expands the discussion here and through the remainder of the book. People with serious mental illness and psychiatric disability are often socially disadvantaged, and this disadvantage may account for many of the barriers to their goals. They may have low incomes, less education, be homeless, or come from culturally disenfranchised groups. Research is unclear whether social disadvantage leads to psychiatric disability or serious mental illness leads to a downward drift into social disadvantage (Draine, Salzer, Culhane, & Hadley, 2002). Direction, however, is beside the point; many of the problems with which people with psychiatric disability struggle may be a function of their social disadvantage more than the symptoms and dysfunctions of their illness.

With disadvantage comes disparity. Many people are unable to partner with competent service providers in order to address the barriers wrought by mental illness blocking their goals. Disadvantaged people in urban settings often lack service options, especially during significant economic recession. Rural settings have a separate set of hurdles that undermine availability and dissemination of services. Compounding these barriers is an absence of services that represent the exigencies of cultural groups like African Americans, Asian Americans, Latinos, and Native Americans. Absence of available and quality services influences patient attitudes about service. They are more pessimistic about possible benefits. Add these concerns to the harmful side effects of medication and psychosocial treatments and it is clear why many people might not pursue services or leave early.

SETTING THE FRAME FOR STIGMA

Stigma begins and grows in a social ethos, a collection of attitudes and beliefs that have evolved out of human history. Modern medicine and health science are a major force for this ethos in the twenty-first century Western world. My goal here was to show that some of what emerged alongside successful health research fueled the stigma that harms people with mental illness. "They cannot take care of themselves. They won't recover. They are dangerous. They are doomed to failure." Common beliefs like these may not have created stigma but clearly are a force for maintaining it.

Unintended outcomes are not the death sentence of psychiatry. Mistakes and corrections are essential to the scientific enterprise. At one time, the best evidence led us to believe the world was flat while the sun revolved around Earth. Galileo's heliocentric universe righted this misdirection. Medicine too has had its share of scientific beliefs—illness represents an imbalance of the four temperaments: phlegmatic, choleric, sanguine, and melancholic—turned on their head by subsequent research. We do not discard current practice because Hippocrates had it wrong. But we also do not insist on old notions in the light of current evidence.

The science of psychiatry is even a bit more challenging than astronomy or medicine. Planets do not interact with astronomers when charting the heavens. There is some objective distance between sick patient and physician in understanding illness. However, the observer and the observed are intimately interlaced in psychology and psychiatry such that neat tactics of objectivity have limits. Hence, perhaps psychiatry compared to the hard sciences is a bit more prone to error in proposing theories that are not wholly borne by independent evidence. Let us learn from these lessons as we now turn our attention to the challenges of mental illness stigma.

2

WHAT IS THE STIGMA OF
MENTAL ILLNESS?

ENTAL ILLNESS STRIKES with a two-edged sword. On one side are the harmful effects of symptoms and disabilities that prevent people from achieving personal goals. On the other are the egregious effects of stigma, the prejudice and discrimination of a community that blocks personal aspirations. Chapter 1 reviewed what research shows to be barriers wrought by psychiatric illness. The chapter also examined how unintended consequences of this research might fan the flames of stigma. In chapter 2, I begin to examine the gist of this book—what is known about stigma and the ways it harms people labeled with mental illness. Psychiatry frames illness as a problem of the individual. Hence, treatment is largely oriented to impacting that person. Stigma is a problem of the community. Resolving it requires targeting where everyone lives, works, and plays.

I begin this chapter by providing a social-psychological model of stigma that focuses on its cognitive constructs and specific functions: stereotypes, prejudice, and discrimination that manifest as public or self-stigma. I then address a social-developmental question: why has stigma emerged in culture as such a harmful force? I seek to illustrate these points by drilling down into the effects of the worst of mental illness stereotypes: dangerousness. Why does viewing people with mental illness as homicidal maniacs endure? This dovetails with an independent but equally egregious set of socially sanctioned stereotypes of behavioral health, that are experienced by people with substance use disorders. This work is governed by recommendations that comprised the National Academy of Sciences report on addressing the stigma of behavioral health.

The second half of this chapter sets the frame for the remainder of the book. How might the stigma of mental illness be erased? This is an especially important focus for social progressives. While this kind of energy is essential for social justice goals such as erasing stigma, its unintended consequences can be dismaying. Scientists have called this the dodo bird effect. I believe it is a different side of the stigma effect. Given these mistakes, the chapter ends with an important question. How do progressives distinguish effective from ineffective anti-stigma strategies? Brief consideration of research to answer this question is discussed.

WHO IS THE STIGMATIZED GROUP?

Because stigma is a social construction, almost any condition can be stigmatized. As a result, there are many groups of people who might be objects of stigma. Jane Elliott demonstrated the seemingly endless breadth of stigmatized conditions with her third-grade class in Riceville, Iowa, the day after Martin Luther King Jr. was assassinated in 1968. She arbitrarily split the class into blue-eyed and brown-eyed students telling the children that blue-eyed classmates were superior. Blue-eyed children were then provided extra food at lunch and more time during recess. Those with blue eyes sat in the front of the classroom while brown-eyed children were relegated to the back. Brown-eyed and blue-eyed children had to drink from separate water fountains. The teacher chastised brown-eyed students when they failed to follow class rules.

Although there was resistance to the rules at first, blue-eyed children soon became disagreeable to their "inferior" classmates. Grades on simple tests were better for blue-eyed children. Brown-eyed children morphed into subservient peers who scored worse on tests. They seemed to isolate themselves from classmates. The next day, Elliott reversed the rules: brown-eyed children were now preferred and blue-eyed students inferior. The ugly face of stigma reversed as well with brown-eyed children dominant and blue-eyed children withdrawn. The exercise had profound impact on the children, teaching them that prejudice and discrimination are arbitrary constructions of an ignorant world. Elliott's work was also insightful for social scientists. It showed what scholars intuitively knew. Almost any condition could be stigmatized. Eye color, handedness, and hair color join those with a more egregious history of stigma: skin color, gender-consistent body features, and indicators of age.

Which conditions, in any historical time, are stigmatized and which are not? Social scientists see this as an empirical question and have crafted ideas like entitativity as a way to explain it. Entitativity is the degree to which the population views any collection of people as a meaningful group. Ethnicity, religion, and gender are all seen as meaningful social entities. African Americans, Christians, and women engender characteristics that the public quickly recognizes. Negative characteristics of the perceived group generate stigma. History illustrates the fluidity of groups defined as stigmatized. Currently, most people do not mindfully split right- versus left-handed people into groups and express preference for one over the other. Left-handedness, however, has been stigmatized for hundreds of years. Some cultures equated the left hand with personal hygiene. Religions including Christianity (Jesus sits at the right hand of God the father) believed right is superior to left. Left-handed people are viewed as less lucky than righties. As result, schools frequently sought to correct mishandedness by requiring left handers to use their right hands.

> I was educated in the USA in Catholic school in the 60s. My left hand was beaten until it was swollen, so I would use my right [sic] hand.
>
> My fourth grade teacher . . . would force me to use my right hand to perform all of my school work. If she caught me using my left hand, I was hit in the head with a dictionary. It turned out that she believed left handers were connected with Satan.
>
> (University of Indiana, 2002)

Most people now realize handedness biases are harmful. Groups like *Anything Left Handed* in the United Kingdom have appeared as supportive and empowering homes for lefties.

Research has shown mental illness to be a meaningful social entity that generates stigmatizing reactions (Rüsch, Corrigan, Wassel et al., 2009a,b).

The public views "the mentally ill" as a cogent group with boundaries that distinguish it from other groups. For example, people with substance use disorders or intellectual disabilities are viewed differently than those with mental illness (Corrigan et al., 2000; Pescosolido et al., 2010; Schomerus et al., 2011; Werner & Shulman, 2015). Each of these groups has specific beliefs that define them.

- People with mental illness are unpredictable and dangerous.
- People with substance use disorders are amoral criminals.
- People with intellectual disabilities are socially stupid and incompetent.

The public makes sense of a stigmatized group as *figure* highlighted against the omnipresent majority, the *ground*: gay versus straight, black versus white, female versus male. Figure is stigmatized while ground is preferred. The ground is a bit more difficult to label for mental illness but for ease of writing, I call it the "normal" majority. Normal, as used here, is absolutely not meant to represent any sense of average or preferred. Normal is not to be valued. Instead, normal is the obverse of the stigmatized construction of mental illness and as such exists only as in terms of that construction. Normal is what the population has called people who do not identify with a history of mental health challenges; they do not perceive themselves as in the group of people with mental health challenges. Normal is the ground against which the figure of mental illness stands.

Advocates believe one way to deal with stigma is for members of a group to stand proudly together against the stigmatizing majority. Accentuate the figure in relation to the ground. Black pride, gay pride, and female pride encourage African Americans, gays, and women to recognize cherished qualities of their group and embrace them in solidarity. The relation between figure and ground vis-à-vis health stigma is more complex. It might seem that solidarity is not a goal for mental illness stigma. After all, isn't the number one goal of being in the mental illness group to get out of it? Through treatment, symptoms are erased and disabilities are replaced so that the person no longer meets diagnostic criteria for that group. Stigma can be dismissed by curing the disease.

Group membership, however, is more than a diagnostic label. Some people, as the result of their illness or treatment or lessons learned from both, identify with the group called mentally ill. It is part of who they are—not a person broken by mental illness but a person who is in recovery from mental illness. This identity is what defines the group, a distinction that leads to an alternative way of defining a group as stigmatized by mental illness. It is a collection of people who are motivated to act against the stigma because of the harm experienced by it. Consider *Sea Change*, a group out of San Francisco whose mission is to address the stigma experienced by women who have had abortions. These are people who are motivated to organize into an advocacy group meant to tear down its harmful effects. Consider the Simon Foundation; their more-than-thirty-year mission is to tackle the stigma experienced by people who have experienced urinary or bowel incontinence. They include people with incontinence who have organized against the stigma.

People with lived experience vote with their feet. This is the most compelling answer to the question, who is the stigmatized group? Because of stigma, they work together over time to act out their mission against the stigma of different conditions. They stand up with their condition, tell their stories, testify to legislators, stuff envelopes, make policy, and raise funds—all trying to stop stigma. They are motivated where motivation is measured by sustained action.

Voting with one's feet is not a trivial mark of motivation. It separates advocacy programs with real energy from those that rest on slacktivism. Slacktivism is defined as a feel-good approach to addressing social injustice with little actual benefit; it has become especially prevalent with the rise of social media. Facebook efforts to speak against an injustice require nothing more than a mouse click. This endorsement is unlikely to generalize to meaningful action. People voting with their feet indicates a motivated group that is likely to sustain energy and resources over time. They use their concerted efforts to make actual behavioral change.

PAN-STIGMATIZED ADVOCACY GROUPS

Some advocates believe that their social justice focus should be more on stigma per se than on the conditions that are stigmatized. The "group" therefore is not a collection of people with specific conditions but all people who are harmed by stigma. The *Rude2Respect* (R2R) program, for example, seeks to change stigma across health conditions. Their website highlights just three of the many stigmatized health conditions in R2R's sights: obesity, hearing loss, and physical disability. R2R's website hosts a challenge wall where people with lived experience assert their message of change (Simon Foundation, 2017).

- "I challenge women to talk about pelvic organ prolapse, to help others recognize that symptoms can be improved with guidance and support." Sher, Wisconsin.
- "I challenge my friends and family to not remark on what beautiful children my husband and I have. We are unable to have children due to a medical condition." Amanda, London.
- "I challenge people to stop assuming how to help me navigate on my crutches." Herman, Montreal.
- "I challenge people to stop shouting at me when they notice I wear a hearing aid." Daniel, North Carolina.

B Stigma-Free takes the pan-stigma agenda further as one program where all isms are erased. They seek to eradicate stigma and prejudice across the breadth of human experience: health, ethnicity, gender, sexual orientation, and much more. *B Stigma-Free* coined the term *cross-identity collaboration* as their working principle. They believe that working together across groups cross-pollinates ideas from differing groups and helps people work better together.

While I salute the intent of pan-stigma programs, I question their efficacy. Many people harmed by the stigma of mental illness are likely to sympathize with ignorant beliefs about people from other stigmatized groups; there is a shared quality to the injustice of stigma. But I believe the motivation of an advocacy group is directed to stigma of a specific condition. The human resource comprising advocacy groups is limited. Efforts extended to other groups are those that cannot address their agenda. Moreover, anti-stigma priorities vary by condition. People with mental illness struggle with the real-world effects of discrimination on work and independent living goals. People with Alzheimer's disease seek independence in a time in their life when many work and independent living goals have been achieved. A pan-agenda will not catch differences like these.

Finally, anti-stigma advocacy groups need financial resources to support their efforts. The pot of monies available from government and private foundations is limited. Hence, advocates for one group are likely to not want to lose resources for their agenda to another group.

INTERSECTIONALITY

The stigmatizing experience is even more complex because many people are harmed by multiple stigmas. Consider Leroy, an African American with mental illness recently released from the county jail. He was homeless prior to his latest jail term and was incarcerated for possession of cocaine. Social scientists call the individual's experience of multiple stigmatized groups *intersectionality* (Crenshaw, Gotanda, Peller, & Thomas, 1995). The idea developed at the intersection of studies on racism and sexism. How is the experience of an African American woman understood? Is she harmed by being black in a white world, female in a male world, or some mix therein? Intersectionality suggests the experience is more than an additive solution.

Stigmatized identity within the individual is experienced changeably. One day Leroy might be sensitive to and harmed by the stigma of mental illness. Another day the stigma related to being an ex-offender is dominant. Social scientists have developed intricate models for explaining how differing identities impact the stigmatized experience of individuals and groups. Intersectionality has several implications for anti-stigma efforts at the level of the group and the individual. First, mental illness stigma in the black community is different than among whites. Hence, programs addressing the stigma of mental illness need to vary by ethnic group.

Second, individual goals for stigma change are driven by the individual. Hence, Leroy needs to be empowered to set the agenda for his stigma change efforts. It might start with an effort to erase the stigma of mental illness but then segue into stigmas related to homelessness and being an ex-offender as Leroy's priorities evolve.

A MODEL OF MENTAL ILLNESS STIGMA

I propose a two-by-four grid in table 2.1 incorporating cognitive and behavioral constructs as one way to make sense of the stigma of mental illness. Social psychologists have a rich body of research that has evolved out of their work, first on ethnicity, but also gender, sexual orientation, and health conditions (Dion, 2002; Herek, 2007; Howarth, 2006). These models have been extended to the stigma of mental illness anchored by three constructs: stereotypes, prejudice, and discrimination. Stigma fundamentally rests on a presumption of difference. Erving Goffman (1963) characterized stigma as "undesired differentness" that results from a mark distinguishing an outgroup from the majority. Blacks are different from whites, gays from straights, young from old. People with psychiatric disability are different from the "normal" majority. Difference as it appears in social exchange is almost always bad and leads to disdain. Blacks are somehow less than whites. People with mental illness are worse than the "normal" majority.

Stereotypes define these differences; they are knowledge structures framed as fact-based beliefs. For example, one widely held belief about Irish

TABLE 2.1 A MATRIX FOR UNDERSTANDING STIGMA: CONSTRUCTS BY TYPOLOGY TO DESCRIBE THE "WHAT" OF STIGMA

		TYPOLOGY			
		PUBLIC STIGMA	SELF-STIGMA	LABEL AVOIDANCE	STRUCTURAL STIGMA
Cognitive	**Prejudice (stereotypes)** dangerous responsible incompetent	"He is dangerous."	"I am unreliable."	Diagnosis of mental illness means "crazy."	Positive personnel actions are suspended.
Behavioral	**Discrimination avoidance/ withdrawal segregation coercion**	Employer refuses to hire person with mental illness.	Person with mental illness does not take on new tasks.	Individual avoids clinics to seek help.	Person with mental illness is not promoted.

Americans is "we are drunken sots who waste family resources so that wife and children live in poverty." Americans learn stereotypes when growing up in our culture; stereotypes are inescapable. Most readers know Irish Americans are drunks. Stereotypes become prejudice when people agree with the belief—"That's right. Irish American men are drunken sots!"—followed by negative emotions and evaluations of the group. "And because they are drunks, they are disgustingly weak men." Discrimination is the behavioral result of prejudice, typically punitive in form and causing loss of rightful opportunity ("I won't hire those drunken Irishmen.") or aversive reactions ("I think Irishmen should be locked up overnight every time they get drunk.").

Research has identified a variety of prejudices and discriminatory behaviors reflecting the stigma of mental illness. Most damning is that of dangerousness, that people labeled with mental illness are unpredictable, violent felons. Stereotypes of dangerousness have such broad and deep effects on people with mental illness that they are dissected later in this chapter. Another stereotype is responsibility, e.g., people with these conditions somehow choose their illness. A third is incompetence, that people with these disorders are unable to fill the roles sought by most peers in their culture. They are unable to work a real job, live in a nice apartment, or enjoy intimate relationships.

TYPES OF STIGMA

The harmful functions of prejudice and discrimination manifest themselves in the four types listed in table 2.1. *Public stigma* occurs when the "normal" majority endorse stereotypes of mental illness and act in a discriminatory manner. It represents what the public does to people known to have mental illness. Three groups of discriminatory behaviors result. First is avoidance and withdrawal; members of the general public avoid people with mental illness in order to escape their violent behavior. Hence, they will not want residential programs for people with mental illnesses in their backyard. They will not want to interact with them at church. Avoidance is especially harmful when acted on by employers and landlords. Prejudiced employers will not hire people with mental illness because they fear physical harm to coworkers. Housing options for individuals with mental illness are limited by stigma. Prejudiced landlords will not rent to people with serious mental illnesses in order to protect their property.

An especially haunting form of discrimination is seen in the primary health care system. Research by Benjamin Druss and colleagues (2000) suggests that people labeled with mental illness are less likely to benefit from the American health care system than people without these labels. The research team examined medical records of more than 100,000 patients in the US Veterans Affairs Health System who presented with symptoms suggesting heart trouble where referral to a specialist was expected. They found that almost 100 percent of veterans presenting with these symptoms, but no known behavioral health disorders, were referred to the coronary care clinic. Only 80 percent of veterans known by the physician to have a substance use disorder were referred. This number fell to 40 percent if the doctor believed the veteran had a mental illness. Two lessons resound. First, stigma and discrimination are no longer vague abstractions but rather issues of life and death. Veterans with mental illness who were not referred for coronary workup experienced worse illness and even death. Second, these were discriminations done by physicians, perhaps the class of people who are most educated about health.

Two other kinds of discriminatory behaviors emerge from the research literature: segregation and coercion. In the past, people with serious mental illnesses were committed to state mental health asylums believing they were incompetent and therefore could not live independently in their community. Although state institutions have downsized greatly, they have been replaced in many states by nursing homes that provide custodial care where people are often relegated to roles of patients expecting to take their medication but not much more. Additionally, absence of independent housing programs has relegated many people with mental illness to the impoverished areas of town to form mental health ghettoes. Both scenarios result in unnecessary segregation of individuals with mental illness from the larger community.

Concerns about dangerousness in a system where services, support, and supervision are sparse have led to coercive interventions. Involuntary commitment to acute inpatient settings is one example. Coercive interventions have also followed people into the community in the form of outpatient commitment and mental health court. I do not mean to suggest these strategies are bad practices per se; mental health court, in particular, may help the individual with mental illness to avoid jail. Still, some strategies can be misused leading to coercive interactions.

Has public stigma improved over the past fifty years? Phelan and colleagues (2000) answered this question by contrasting the extent to which the public believes people with mental illness are dangerous in 1996 with similar data from 1956 (see figure 2.1). Hoping that public knowledge about mental illness has improved during those forty years, one might expect the rate of endorsing these stereotypes to halve, perhaps from 40 to 20 percent. The results, however, were the reverse. Twice the number of people in 1996 compared to 1956 believed people with mental illness are dangerous. The research was repeated in 2006 with, once again, about 40 percent of the American public agreeing that people with mental illness are dangerous (Pescosolido et al., 2010). These data reflecting American opinions are echoed by meta-analyses of population studies done around the world (Schomerus et al., 2011); meta-analysis is a research strategy where statistical findings from multiple studies are collapsed into a mega summary of results. The scientists in this study found acceptance of people labeled with

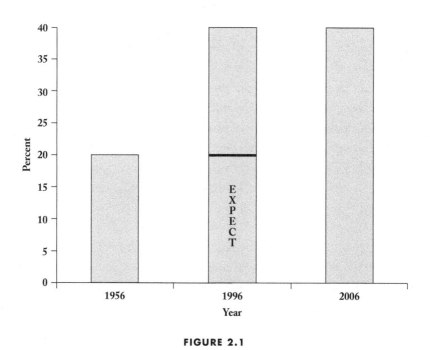

FIGURE 2.1

Change in population beliefs about the dangerousness of people with mental illness.

schizophrenia has gotten notably worse. People do not want neighbors or coworkers with mental illness. Keep these sobering findings foremost in mind; stigma is getting worse despite the world seeming to be more educated about mental illness.

Self-stigma is a second type of stigma that occurs when people internalize prejudice ("I am mentally ill so I must be incompetent.") and discriminate against themselves ("I am not going to try to get a good job because I can't handle it."). If it is hard enough to deal with the stress and depression of mental illness, people must also deal with the shame that occurs from the publicly perceived weakness. Internalizing stigma hurts self-esteem ("I am not worthy.") and lessens self-efficacy ("I am not able.") leading to a "why try" effect. "Why should I try to get a job? I am not good enough." "Why try to live independently? I am unable." There is a terrible irony to the self-stigma of mental illness. It is already troubling to deal with the distress and sadness of mental illness that undermines one's sense of self-worth. On top of that, people must be shamed into the closet because of unjust stereotypes.

Label avoidance is the third type of stigma. To understand label avoidance, the reader needs to first understand the varied character of stigma. In his classic discourse, Erving Goffman (1963) distinguished stigma that results from obvious versus hidden marks. Obvious stigma occurs when marks causing prejudice and discrimination are readily observable: skin color for racism, body differences for sexism, and wheel chairs for the stigma of physical disability. There are no manifest cues that absolutely mark someone as suggesting mental illness. Sure, some people with mental illness are disheveled, but so are many homeless individuals. Some people with mental illness act oddly in public but so do those we might call eccentric. The mark that signals mental illness is the label. "Karen has schizophrenia." And labels become public when the person is known to visit a mental health service. "Hey, that's Karen coming out of that psychiatrist's office. She must be nuts!" Hence, one way to avoid stigma is to avoid mental health services from which labels are obtained. Epidemiological research shows the harmful effects of label avoidance. As many as one-third to half of people challenged by mental illness will not seek out services in times of need (Mojtabai et al., 2011). This applies across diagnoses, for people with serious disorders such as schizophrenia to the most benign of problems that might result from short-term stress. In addition, about half of people who do seek out services will drop out early (Olfson et al., 2009).

Oftentimes people do not get treatment because appropriate services are lacking. Absence of appropriate services is the fourth type, *structural stigma*. The idea of structural stigmas evolved from the field of sociology and manifests in two ways: (1) policies of private and governmental institutions that intentionally restrict the opportunities of people with mental illnesses, and (2) policies that yield unintended consequences that hinder the options of people with mental illness (Pincus, 1999). Intentional structural discrimination manifests itself as rules, policies, and procedures of private and public entities in positions of power that purposefully restrict the rights and opportunities of minority groups. Jim Crow laws from the nineteenth and early twentieth centuries are examples of intended structural discrimination. Largely enacted by southern states, these laws restricted African American rights in employment, education, and public accommodation. There are similar examples in mental health such as statutes that restrict a person's parental rights because of past history of mental illness. One of the errors of these laws is assuming that a person with schizophrenia two years ago will continue to be disabled by the illness today. Legislative failure to prioritize mental health services, especially interventions that promote recovery-based interventions, is another example of structural stigma.

There are also public and private sector policies whose consequences restrict the opportunities of minority groups in unintended ways, instances where discrimination seemingly results without conscious effort. Pincus (1999) provided a useful example. Prestigious universities often use the SAT to limit admission offers to students with the highest scores. Given that African American and Latino students typically score lower than whites on these tests, universities that rely on the SAT likely prevent a disproportionate number of students of color from receiving an education at their institution. In terms of mental illness, less money is allocated to research and treatment on psychiatric illness than other health disorders; illnesses like cancer and heart disease dominate the American public health agenda even though the World Health Organization (Sayers, 2001) showed mental illnesses and substance use disorders are equally or even more disabling. In addition, many psychiatrists and other mental health professionals opt out of the public system serving people with the most serious psychiatric disorders. Salaries and benefits are better in private health systems that treat relatively benign illnesses like adjustment disorders or relational problems.

Important to note is that structural stigma is not really discussed in more detail in this book. In part, this reflects a failure of psychologists like me who have failed to explain the phenomenon more fully. Structural stigma is more often examined by sociologists and hence has been mostly outside my scope. In addition, approaches to changing structural stigma are largely undeveloped. The lesson here is the need for future work in this appropriate arena.

WHAT SIGNALS STEREOTYPES?

The general public infers mental illness from four cues: psychiatric symptoms, social skills deficits, poor physical appearance, and labels. Many of the symptoms of severe mental illness—inappropriate affect, bizarre behavior, language irregularities, and talking to oneself aloud—are manifest indicators of psychiatric illness that frighten the public. Symptoms like these may produce stigmatizing reactions. Moreover, poor social skills that are a function of psychiatric illness also lead to stigmatizing reactions. Deficits in eye contact, body language, and choice of discussion topics potentially mark a person as "mentally ill" and lead to stigmatizing attitudes. Personal appearance may also lead to stigmatizing attitudes. In particular, diminished physical attractiveness and personal hygiene may be manifest indicators of mental illness leading to stereotypic responses from one's community; e.g., "that unkempt person on the park bench must be a mental patient."

Note, however, the potential for misattributing someone as "mentally ill" based on these first three signals. What might be eccentric behavior that is not characteristic of a psychiatric disorder (e.g., the musician singing aloud a piece from an upcoming concert) could be misunderstood as mental illness. Fewer social skills may represent a shy person rather than mental illness. Physical appearance may also lead to false positives about judging someone as "mentally ill." Many street people with slovenly appearance are believed to be "mentally ill" when, in actuality, they are just poor and homeless. Just as these three signs may yield false positives, so the absence of these signs will lead to false negatives. Many people are able to conceal their experiences with mental illness without those around them being aware. Goffman (1963) more fully developed this point when he distinguished between what might be called obvious and hidden stigma. The former occurs when people have a mark that is readily perceivable. Examples of the obvious group include persons from a cultural minority with an apparent physical trait that leads them to believe that their differences are obvious to the public; e.g., Africans have dark skin. Persons with hidden stigma, on the other hand, can conceal their condition; they have no readily observable mark that identifies them as part of a stigmatized group. For example, one's sexual orientation cannot be discerned by an obvious cue. The public frequently cannot determine whether a person is "mentally ill" by merely looking at him or her. Only in those cases where the person is acutely ill and floridly psychotic might he or she be accurately identified as "mentally ill."

Juxtaposing concerns about false positives with the idea that the stigma of mental illness may be hidden begs the question, what, then, is the definite mark that leads to stigmatizing responses? Several carefully constructed studies suggest labels as a key signal leading to stereotypes, prejudice, and discrimination. People who are known as "mentally ill" will likely be the victim of mental illness stigma. Labels can be obtained in various ways: others can tag people with a label (a psychiatrist can inform someone that Ms. X is mentally ill), individuals can label themselves (a person can decide to introduce himself as a psychiatric survivor), or labels can be obtained by association (a person observed coming out of a psychologist's office may be assumed to be mentally ill).

AFFIRMING ATTITUDES AND BEHAVIOR

Erasing the prejudice and discrimination of mental illness is not sufficient. They need to be replaced with affirming attitudes and behaviors. Soon after Lyndon Johnson passed the civil rights law meant to erase American racism in 1964, he said, "You do not wipe away the scars of centuries by saying: Now you are free to go where you want, and do as you desire, and choose the leaders you please." Civil rights only are achieved by promoting affirmative action. Erasing the hurtful effects of the prejudice and discrimination of mental illness is not enough; they need to be replaced by affirming attitudes and behaviors. Affirming attitudes include ideas of recovery and self-determination. We know anti-stigma efforts are successful when the public endorses processes of recovery—that the human story, even for those with the most serious of mental illnesses, is one of hope and achievement. Regardless of symptoms and disabilities, everyone is capable of aspirations in vocation, independent living, and relationships, goals that can be attained with appropriate support. Anti-stigma agenda are also impactful when the public recognizes the primacy of self-determination, that people with mental illness decide for themselves personal goals and ways to achieve these goals.

Attitudes, of course, are never enough. Anti-stigma effort also demands affirming behavior. Title I of the Americans with Disabilities Act (ADA, 1990) is a powerful example. The ADA requires employers to provide reasonable accommodations to employees with disabilities. Reasonable accommodations are modifications in settings and operations in which work gets done so people with disabilities can do their jobs competently. A familiar example would be changes in a physical plant so people using wheelchairs can navigate the facility. Reasonable accommodations extend beyond the workplace to provide accessibility and utility of most public accommodations. Hence, people with physical disabilities expect public facilities to be fully available to them.

The stigma of mental illness is erased when reasonable accommodations become widespread for those with psychiatric disabilities. This has by no means been easy. George H. W. Bush signed the ADA to much acclaim from the disability community in 1990. It was in place for more than five years before the government asserted its relevance for those with psychiatric disability. The Equal Employment Opportunity Commission released an executive order stating that the ADA does apply to those with psychiatric disorders and directing government agencies to act accordingly. Despite this directive, reasonable accommodations for psychiatric disability have been slow to arrive perhaps because of intrinsic differences between physical and mental health disabilities. Physical disabilities are obvious as are accommodations such as bigger elevators and doors for wheelchair access. Accommodations for psychiatric disabilities are harder to perceive. Perhaps first among accommodations are support specialists for people wanting them. These are job coaches who accompany people with psychiatric disabilities to work each day, helping them plan that day's tasks. Housing coaches meet people at their home regularly to address practical chores of daily living. Stigma has been trumped when these accommodations are provided freely within one's community.

Affirmative behaviors and reasonable accommodations are not charity; they are the rightful expectations of people with disabilities. The Civil Rights Act was passed in 1964 to make sure people of color have the same chances as the white majority. The ADA provides similar assurances. It is absurd to argue that affirmative behaviors provide unfair advantage to the person with disabilities. Reasonable accommodations level the playing field. Accommodations are not unlimited. The ADA specifies caps to reasonable accommodations, requests that cause "undue hardship" on employers and their business. Many nine-to-five offices, for example, might find it difficult for workers to come in at midnight to do their work. However, experience suggests that the ADA and reasonable accommodations are not viewed as intrusive or demanding by most employers. Bosses want their workers to be successful, in part, because employers are reasonable human beings, and in part because accommodations are wise policy. Businesses fail when they terminate and then need to train a new batch of employees.

EMPOWERMENT

The obverse of self-stigma is personal empowerment. People with mental illness who view themselves as worthy and believe their goals are achievable are able to suppress the harmful effects of self-stigma. Empowerment includes four components (Rogers, Chamberlin, Ellison, & Crean, 1997): self-efficacy and self-esteem, which include positive attitudes about oneself and feelings of accomplishment; optimism, beliefs that a person can accomplish their goals; community activism, people who work together have greater impact on their community; and righteous anger, making waves will help to move the discussion forward.

FROM WHENCE COMES STIGMA?

How come stigmas occur and endure? In particular, how come the public creates stereotypes about those labeled with mental illness that lead to discrimination? Two reasons emerge: kernel of truth and justification of the status quo.

KERNEL OF TRUTH

From this perspective, what is called mental illness stigma is normal reaction to bizarre behavior of people with psychiatric illness. Hence, stigma is not a social injustice, in the sense of misperceiving a group. In 1980, a National Institute of Mental Health workshop chose not to include "stigma" in its title because they believed the term is inappropriate if "one is referring to negative attitudes induced by manifestations of psychiatric illness" (Rabkin, Muhlin, & Cohen, 1984, p. 327). In other words, negative attitudes make sense as a normal response to the symptoms of mental illness. Stigma as normal echoes arguments of 1970s' sociology (Gove, 1975); namely, societal reactions to individuals with mental illness are the natural response to psychiatric symptoms rather than biased expectations activated by some other source of stigma like labels. While Gove does not deny that labels generate negative reactions, he discounts their importance in the "causation" and persistence of psychiatric stigma. He suggests having been labeled a "former mental patient" does not meaningfully harm opportunities in the community.

Research has put Gove to the test in twelve studies where research participants were exposed to stigma-consistent behavior (talking to self or believing in alien possession) or a stigmatizing label (that person is schizophrenic) (see review by Link, 1987). Some research suggests that rejection experienced by individuals with mental illness results from their deviant behavior rather than stigmatized label. Ten of twelve studies showed that aberrant behavior had a statistically significant and more potent effect than labels on subsequent prejudice and discrimination. However, Link (1987) also found that people with mental illness experience discrimination regardless of their behavior. In their work, the researchers observed objectionable behavior leading to stigma. But the authors also noted that prejudice and discrimination activated by the label—by just calling someone schizophrenic—was as important, if not more so, than behavior in determining rejection. Some people who act eccentrically in the community will be viewed in a stigmatizing way and that might make sense. However, when that behavior, or any kind of eccentric activity, is labeled as mentally ill, then stigma skyrockets.

The "normal response" hypothesis was alternatively framed in social psychological research as a kernel of truth (Allport, 1979). Put simply, if groups possess real and objective differences, then stereotypes reflecting group differences logically follow. Hence, if people with mental illness are, in fact, more bizarre, dangerous, incompetent, and irresponsible than the "normal" majority, it is reasonable that these traits are attributed to the category of mental illness. Assessment of the kernel of truth hypothesis, therefore, is a matter of assessing "stereotype accuracy." Examples are apparent in perceptions of a variety of social groups. Professional basketball players are stereotyped as tall, which is mostly confirmed. But stereotype accuracy is limited to physical attributes. More than half a century ago, Vinacke (1949) uncovered reported stereotype accuracy in perceptions of Japanese, Chinese, white, Korean, Filipino, Hawaiian, Samoan, and African American students at the University of Hawaii. His research suggested, for example, that students "accurately" perceived Hawaiians as musical and easygoing.

Most social scientists now question accuracy of stereotyped perceptions; history is filled with inaccurate stereotypes that only justify pernicious forms of prejudice and discrimination. Chinese were viewed as "sly" and "deceitful." Armenian laborers were stereotyped as "dishonest," "deceitful," and "troublemakers." Especially egregious among these was the assertion that blacks were intellectually inferior. This view was fanned by writings of Berkeley psychologist Arthur Jensen (1969) that suggested IQ is largely determined by genetics thereby explaining why people of African races were less successful academically. Most readers will likely cringe at these racist notions clothed in academic writings. In case there might be doubt, objective assessments of group characteristics consistently fail to confirm the validity of these stereotypes. Performance of blacks on standardized achievement tests matches that of similar white Americans when blacks take these tests under conditions that minimize stereotype threat (Steele & Aronson, 1995). Support for kernel of truth is absent.

JUSTIFICATION OF THE STATUS QUO

An alternative view gaining research support is that stereotypes and discrimination evolve because they psychologically protect people and their groups. Stigma provides justification for a status quo that represents disparities among groups. Three kinds of justification have been identified: ego justification, group justification, and system justification. Psychoanalysts were among the first to write clearly about ego justification; namely, the self is protected when internal conflicts are projected onto stigmatized groups (Bettleheim & Janowitz, 1964). Instead of thinking "I" am not competent, individuals buffer self-image against interpersonal failings by viewing people with mental illness (among the many possible stigmatized groups) as not socially skilled. Despite its intellectual appeal and omnipresence in the clinical literature, little empirical evidence has been found to support ego justification. Alternatively, stigma and stereotypes may serve a self-protective function that does not have psychodynamic implications. The goals of stigma may be to avoid potential threat to one's body or psychological self (Biernat & Dovidio, 2000). There is some research support here. Studies showed that people are more likely to endorse out-group stereotypes when their self-image had been undermined during a self-affirmation task (Fein & Spencer, 1997; Spencer, Fein, Wolfe, Fong, & Dunn, 1998). Although more supportive of self-justification as a model, it still fails to explain the essential question of this chapter: why does mental illness stigma take the specific forms known in the Western world? Why are people with mental illness viewed as dangerous and incompetent rather than, for example, ugly and lazy? This limitation is more fully explained after reviewing research on group-justification models.

Other research argued that group, and not individual, is the appropriate level for understanding status quo justification (Tajfel, 1981). The motivation for group justification is to support the goals of one's in-group. For example, specific stereotypes about a minority out-group serve to frame the majority in a positive light. "All members of the majority are hardworking; out-group minorities are lazy!" Individuals endorse stereotypes as ways of justifying actions of others with whom they closely identify. There is substantial research that supports these assertions (Abrams & Hogg, 1988). In-group bias is significantly stronger when in-group membership is salient. Moreover, higher status groups seem to show more in-group bias on relevant attributes (i.e., those characteristics most important to the group) while lower status groups exhibit more in-group bias on less-relevant attributes. Still, group justification as explanation for mental illness stigma is problematic. What exactly is the in-group against which people with mental illness are contrasted? The "normal" in-group is a default category that only gains definition in the absence of mental illness. Hence, there is no readily apparent source of in-group motivation to drive system justification.

Jost and colleagues (1999) identified an even broader target for justification (beyond the self or group) arguing that stereotypes and prejudice develop to confirm the *system*. Once a set of events produces specific social relationships, whether by historical accident, biological derivation, public policy, or individual intention, resulting arrangements are explained and justified simply because they exist. These justifications seem to evolve over time as the result of historic, economic, or social forces. There are interesting examples of system justification. Because of historical events in the sixteenth and seventeenth centuries, blacks were slaves and whites were masters. The system explains this difference post hoc by stereotyping contemporary blacks as less competent and industrious. Women are able to bear children; men are not. Hence, women are viewed as the caretakers and men the workers and business agents. Women are characterized as nurturing while men are viewed as autonomous.

How might system justification account for mental illness stereotypes? During the Middle Ages, people with mental illness were locked away in prisons. Protection of the public from dangerous people was primary. Beginning in the nineteenth century, prisons were replaced with asylums and hospitals. People are now viewed as incompetent and in need of guardians. Since the deinstitutionalization that began in the 1960s, growing numbers of individuals with mental illness are again ending up in prisons and jails. This trend leads to the popular notion that people with mental illness are dangerous and unable to care for themselves.

System justification suggests that stereotypes require knowledge of past history. The general public must remember slavery to understand a system justification for it. Hence, people need to recognize the historical role of institutionalization to systemically justify mental illness stereotypes. Does this mean the impact of system justification is limited in people who lack historical knowledge? Not necessarily. System justification probably has its greater impetus from contemporary social phenomena that reflect past history. System justifications of African Americans are more likely to arise from obvious social and economic injustices between the races, injustices that have their roots in slavery and its immediate aftermath. In a similar manner, justifications for mental illness may come from the obvious institutions that suggest people with mental illness need to be controlled, e.g., state hospitals and prisons. Note that, in both cases, the news media and entertainment industry have a central role in informing the public about the status quo.

THE STIGMA OF DANGEROUSNESS

Dangerousness is the worst stereotype of mental illness leading to significant public and self-discrimination. How come it is a virulent force in society? Some believe stigma about dangerousness is a reflection of real world experience and therefore reflects a kernel of truth. Others argue that titillating media portrayals of people with mental illness as violent, especially in the entertainment industry, contribute to widespread misperceptions of violence and mental illness. What does research show? Advocates from the Treatment Advocacy Center (TAC) and the American Enterprise Institute (AEI) cite research to support their beliefs about mental illness and dangerousness. The TAC, for example, estimated that persons with serious mental illness commit about 1,000 homicides per year in the United States in a twenty-year span (TAC, 2002). The AEI cited a study that found 300 inpatients of California's State Hospital in 1975 committed violent crimes at a rate that was ten times higher than the general population (Satel, 1998). This has led to forcefully worded calls for greater mental health resources to keep untreated psychiatric patients off the streets and away from hurting others.

Other research groups have criticized interpretations of data that suggest people with mental illness are more dangerous than comparable groups in the population (Bonovitz & Bonovitz, 1981; Link, Andrews, & Cullen, 1992; Teplin, 1983, 1984; Steadman, Cocozza, & Melick, 1978; Wahl, 1995). Four rejoinders emerged. First, there are general versus specific effects in research on mental illness stigma that need to be distinguished in TAC and AEI summaries. The public seems to generally stigmatize all people labeled mentally ill and then specifically stigmatize those with more serious mental illnesses like psychoses beyond the baseline label. Yet, the TAC and AEI suggest that *all* people with a mental illness diagnosis are potentially dangerous. They fail to identify specific symptoms or disabilities resulting from mental illness that cause violence.

Second, the TAC and AEI simplistically conclude that untreated mental illness leads to murder. However, the relationship between mental illness and violence is quite complex, often explained by other relationships. Consider, for example, that the mental illness label is associated with demographic characteristics that have stronger demonstrated ties to violence, that people committing violent crimes are viewed more frequently as mentally ill because of the psychiatrization of criminal behavior, and that people with mental illness are more likely to be arrested for "offending" behaviors than are people without mental illness who commit these behaviors (Teplin, 1984). Third, TAC and AEC generalize from samples of people with mental illness who are in crises (either acutely ill requiring hospitalization, or police involvement because of a violent act) to the entire population of people with mental illness. Extrapolating statistics from criminal records to estimate dangerousness in the population of people with mental illness is not valid. Doing so is parallel to determining the dangerousness of ethnic groups by means of court records rather than probability samples of the population.

Fourth, high rate of news stories depicting people with mental illness as dangerous does not accurately reflect the level of violence among people with psychiatric disorders, although it does demonstrate how the media (re) produces society's fascination with crime in any group (Wahl, 1995). Consider, for example, research findings that people of color are overrepresented as dangerous in the news media. Research does provide evidence for a link between mental illness and dangerousness but the relationship is a murky one. As a result, the National Stigma Clearinghouse partnered with the MacArthur Research Network on Mental Health and the Law to develop a consensus statement that honestly reflects the empirical research findings seeking to contextualize them socially and politically (Monahan & Arnold, 1996). The forty-one researchers, service providers, and consumer advocates who signed the consensus statement agreed on three points:

- Results of several large-scale studies suggest that mental illness is *weakly* associated with violence.
- In spite of these findings, the public perceives a *strong* link to exist between mental illness and dangerousness; as a result, individuals with mental illness and their families experience high levels of stigma.
- Resolving this injustice requires eliminating the stigma and discrimination as well as providing quality treatments to individuals with mental illness.

Despite growing evidence of the disconnect between dangerousness and stigma, misguided advocates have sought to promote policy by propagating the connection. In an October 2015 exchange with ABC News's George Stephanopoulos about gun violence, Donald Trump said, "This isn't guns. This is about, really, mental illness." Congressman Tim Murphy (R-Ohio) was the 2017 lead in a government overhaul of federal policy toward mental health care. At the time, he wore a button that said, "Treatment before tragedy." Finally, clothing designer Kenneth Cole put up billboards meant to promote gun control in 2015. One in New York City read, "Over 40 mill Americans suffer from mental illness. SOME can access care. ALL can access guns." These insidious messages add to news stories and heighten stereotypes about mental illness and dangerousness.

STIGMA BY ASSOCIATION

Family members and friends are also impacted by public stigma. Goffman (1963) called this courtesy stigma—prejudice and discrimination extended to a group by virtue of their relationship with a stigmatized other. Studies have found that parents and siblings of some disabled children, spouses or other partners, as well as other family caregivers, report feeling stigmatized to some degree, and work to manage their self- and public identities in various ways (Moses, 2014). Family members report being victimized by

I found myself on public radio in the United States and Canada three times in the twenty-four-month period beginning January 2011. During that time, Jared Loughner shot Congresswoman Gabrielle Giffords and killed six others in Tucson. James Holmes murdered twelve moviegoers in Aurora, Colorado, watching the latest *Batman* movie. Adam Lanza killed twenty-six, including twenty children, in a Newtown, Connecticut, elementary school. In each case, radio interviewers wanted me to address the apparent link between mental illness and violence. I typically cited evidence that makes up the consensus statement above and expressed concerns about these stories and stigma. People with mental illness were generally NOT likely to be violent and dangerous. But I eventually became worn down by the stories, the overwhelming sadness of these senseless crimes leading to unspeakable tragedy. Accurate summaries of data about inaccurate public perceptions of mental illness felt hollow in this deeply painful need to understand sins against humanity. Then I was reminded of the seminal paper by Bernard Weiner (Weiner & Wright, 1993), *On Sin Versus Sickness*, as explanations of the unspeakable. Weiner believed that humans have a fundamental need to understand why things happen. Who, for example, is responsible for the baseball team winning the championship? Why did Ajax Corporation report an uptick in fourth-quarter sales? How come students at Washington School were falling behind in reading scores? Why did these god-awful shootings occur?

Extrapolating on Weiner, I opined in one interview about the value of sin or sickness for explaining these god-awful shootings. Through most of the past two thousand years, people explained the inexplicable in terms of sin. People committed senseless crimes because they were evil. There was strange solace in conclusions like these because investment in religion seemed to be a way to vanquish the unspeakable. Explanations resting on sin fell to the curb in the age of reason. What used to be left to priests and religious scholars now is the purview of science. Sin was no longer a legitimate answer to horrible acts. Mental illness emerged in the vacuum. We no longer can find answers in the bible, so instead, we look to the DSM.

(continued)

I wondered whether the expulsion of religion was shortsighted and blaming psychiatry is wrong, not just factually but also morally. I hedge this with a personal irony. Although I am a lifelong and Jesuit-trained Catholic, I am no expert on matters of theology. I am expert in social science. Still, I thought explanations of why Jared Loughner, James Holmes, and Adam Lanza did their crimes might be advanced by reintroducing religion to the discussion. Perhaps they did these things not because they are mentally ill but because they are evil. I admittedly said this on the radio with trepidation given that explanations of mental illness have been tainted by sin for centuries. But omitting the consideration for the shooters may leave out an important consideration.

By the way, I received a phone call soon after one of the radio interviews from the National Rifle Association. I was asked on that interview whether I thought people with mental illness should be withheld gun rights. "I do not believe mental illness per se make anyone a better or worse gun owner," that even people with psychoses are able to conduct themselves responsibly most of the time. Even people with psychoses are not always out of touch with reality. So if guns were a Second Amendment right, then citizens with mental illness should be able to enjoy the amendment. Hearing this, the NRA caller invited me to a press conference where I might share that view. "But you missed the first half of my response," I responded. I had told the reporter that I thought "no one should have guns, that the sadness of senseless crimes would be cut exponentially when free access to guns ended in the U.S. altogether."

stereotypes ("The mom must have caused the person to be sick"), leading to discrimination ("people who shun neighbors with children with serious mental illness"). This can also lead to self-stigma: "I must be a bad parent because my child ended up on the psych ward." Some may experience shame, blame, or contamination because of their relationship with relatives identified with mental illness. A family member's role vis-à-vis the "marked" family member—parent, child, sibling, or spouse—relates to the nature and extent of stigma he or she experiences. Parents are typically blamed for causing the stigmatized condition; siblings are viewed as genetically contaminated and possibly blamed for failing to help manage the condition; spouses may also be blamed for poor illness management, as well as possibly degraded based on their voluntary association with the marked individual; and children are often assumed to be genetically and/or psychologically contaminated by the parent's condition, which renders them as "damaged goods."

Stigma may also extend to providers of mental health care, exacerbating public stigma and increasing the likelihood that people will not seek services. A comprehensive review of more than 500 studies suggests the public endorses varied stereotypes about psychiatry and psychiatrists (Sartorius et al., 2010). The practice of psychiatry is often viewed by the public as ineffective or possibly harmful, by medical students as low status, by patients as failing to target essential problems, and by the media as a discipline without true scholarship. Psychiatrists are frequently viewed in a similar negative light. The public views psychiatrists as low status physicians who rely too much on medication. Medical students endorse the idea that psychiatrists "must be crazy." Patient attitudes are often ambivalent with some sincerely grateful for the efforts of their psychiatrists while others view them as controlling and distracted. The media represents psychiatrists as mad doctors, super healers, or exploitive.

I must admit that prioritizing psychiatrist stigma may undermine psychiatry's moral authority in an argument where it had been noticeably missing. At best, posing psychiatrist stigma distracts from the core of the injustice—its harm on people with serious mental illnesses. At worst, it muddies psychiatry's role in promoting recovery. Consider two historical examples. For thousands of years people with leprosy were chased out of their homes into colonies of shame and deprivation. Good people often stepped up to care for those with leprosy, typically suffering the same kind of social opprobrium as those with the disease. Alternatively, the first 250 years of Europe's history in the New World were a time when Africans were brutalized as slaves. Caucasians of conscience spoke out about this moral plague, some working in the Underground Railroad, offering refuge and nourishment to slaves who were fleeing north. The freedom riders risked arrest, jail, and the murderous rage of neighbors. It is hard to focus on the unjust discrimination of carers in leper colonies or freedom fighters on the Underground Railroad, viewing both as a preposterous diversion. Perhaps our comparison is overstated. But then using the stigma of mental illness to describe the woes of psychiatry may be exaggerated. Psychiatrist stigma might gain legitimacy if it had the support of grassroots advocates with serious mental illnesses, those leading the charge against mental illness stigma.

THE STIGMA OF PEOPLE WITH SUBSTANCE USE DISORDERS

Substance use disorders (SUDs) have been lurking in the background of the discussion thus far on mental health and stigma. How does the prejudice and discrimination of SUDs compare to mental illness? While there are many similarities, there is a fundamental difference between the two. The stigma of SUDs is socially, politically, and legally sanctioned. As a result, what seems to be an easy mantra of the stigma movement for mental health—stop it—is muddied for addiction. Consider these three examples.

1. **Discrimination against people with addictions is legal**. Although the justice system often concerns itself with the role of mental illness in criminal guilt and fitness to stand trial, it mostly protects the civil rights of people with serious mental illness—much less so for people with SUDs. Use of controlled substances, including cocaine, opioids, and some medications such as amphetamines and barbiturates, is illegal in most jurisdictions. Penalties for illicit use can vary from monetary fines to extended prison terms. Even more, socially benign substances such as alcohol and tobacco are legally controlled; for example, people under age 18 are not permitted to purchase or use these substances. In the work setting, supervisors can reprimand employees found to be under the influence of alcohol or other psychoactive substances at work.

This kind of stigma is worsened by criminalization by conflating drug use with felonious behavior. Pairing criminal behavior with addiction got a significant boost with the launch of the 1970s war on drugs by the Nixon administration. The war's effects were tragic; one in every 136 adults was incarcerated for drug possession in 2005 (Pew Charitable Trust, 2005).

Although public sentiment about criminalizing drugs waned (for example, the U.S. Department of Justice during the Obama administration called for criminal deinstitutionalization and alternatives to incarceration through the "Second Chance Act"), research shows people who endorse criminal penalties for drug use still endorse the stigma of people labeled with SUD (West, Yanos, & Mulay, 2014).

The stigma of SUD also impacts interpretations of civil law; consider, for example, the reasonable accommodations clause of the ADA. Although reasonable accommodations require job settings to be improved so people with disabilities—including those that result from serious mental illness—successfully complete work-related duties, protections for addictions are comparatively limited. Individuals with addictions do qualify for ADA protections if successfully treated and no longer engaged in illegal use of drugs or currently engaged in a treatment program and not using illegal drugs. Relapse leads to trouble, however. Employers are not violating these acts when disciplining employees—including discharge or denying promotions—currently engaged in illegal use of drugs. The ADA does not falter for people with mental illness who experience recurring symptoms.

2. Stigma is used to promote prevention. Stigma is purposefully incorporated into health communication strategies to promote substance use prevention in two ways. (1) Stress the criminal-addiction connection. Health campaigns have purposefully paired drug use with illegal activity to decrease addiction. Mothers Against Drunk Driving builds much of its public awareness campaign by framing alcohol and drug use in terms of horrific car accidents. The 2002 Super Bowl game compared drug use to terrorism by connecting illegal drug buys to extremists who operate the narco-market beneath it. (2) Public service announcements promote prevention by tying drug use to poor health (Guttman & Salmon, 2004), an especially popular approach for youth programs. The United Nations released a thirty-second PSA in 2010 that followed four young people whose health deteriorates as they use drugs. The 2014 Worlds AIDS campaign targeted fifteen- to twenty-four-year-olds by tying drug use to contracting HIV.

3. Some interventions may worsen self-stigma. Twelve-step programs address SUDs by encouraging members to recognize their absence of power vis-à-vis addictions, admit character defects that result from this powerlessness, and make amends to those they have wronged. This corresponds with disease models that frame people as unable to control substance use because of biological predispositions, a view that may unintentionally promote self-stigma. In mental illness research, self-stigma is often found to be an unintended effect of presenting disease models, often diminishing feelings of self-worth among people. As discussed in chapter 1, recovery models offset these effects from two different vantage points: outcome and process. Outcome models describe recovery as a state where symptoms are remitted, disabilities overcome, and goals achieved. Process models view recovery as a journey described by hope where people pursue personally defined goals regardless of symptoms and disabilities. Recovery reintroduced hope and optimism into discussion of serious mental illnesses, in the process becoming a fundamental tool in tearing down the stigma of mental illness.

Definitions of recovery from addictions are a bit more complex. Recovery is a continuum for mental illness while it is often presented as a clear end state—abstinence—for disease models of addiction. People with SUDs who fail to abstain may promote self-stigma. Although recovery from mental illness is grounded in hope, recovery from addiction sometimes begins with hopelessness and hitting bottom. Recovery from addictions, according to this perspective, only occurs when people recognize their powerlessness in the face of substances.

This sense of powerlessness suggests different perspectives on self-determination. Fundamental to mental health are systems that empower people to define life goals for themselves and then select interventions that help them achieve those goals. Self-determination may be tempered by twelve-step and other addiction programs with concerns about impulsivity where people are warned not to be fooled by aspirations given past failures from substance use.

IMPLICATIONS FOR ERASING THE STIGMA

Rarely are mental health and policy advocates derailed by misunderstanding the goal. Not so for addictions. Because some stigmas are legally or socially sanctioned, changing them is a much more complex task. Criminalizing addiction might be stigmatizing, but no easy consensus will be found in decreasing stigma by breaking the connection between SUDs and crime. Using stigma to promote prevention might seem contrary to public health intentions, but we doubt activists will think this tool should be eliminated. Unlike mental health, the stigma of addiction does not target an irrefutable goal for social advocates.

One benefit of addiction stigma is to reduce substance use. Many might consider it acceptable to endorse stigma should this purpose be achieved. But we have to ask, is it really acceptable to use stigma as a public health tool? And does stigma in fact reduce substance use, or does it, as mounting evidence suggests, cause more harm than good? And further, how can substance use problems be better managed without stigma, without devaluation, discrimination, and exclusion of persons with addictions? As advocates of social change, these are exquisitely complex questions that advocates, providers, and people with lived experience need to consider with the benefit of empirical research.

Differences in stigmas might suggest substance use is socially worse than mental illness. After all, substance abuse is illegal and immoral. This kind of comparison is illegitimate and harmful. Advocates need to make sure they do not unintentionally worsen the stigma of substance use when trying to erase the stigma of mental illness.

"Well at least people with mental illness are not as bad as substance abusers!"

It would be like reducing racism by saying, "at least blacks are not as bad as Latinos who sneak into our country and steal our jobs!"

We have wandered into the area of stigma change with this discussion. In the next section, approaches to erasing the stigma of mental illness are more carefully examined.

Given that stigma varies by type (e.g., public and self-stigma, label avoidance, and structural stigma), I believe stigma change varies by conceptual level as well. Work has mostly examined ways to impact the harmful effects of public stigma and self-stigma. Specific strategies for both are briefly reviewed here. The remainder of the book dissects relative benefits as well as unintended consequences of each.

The Opioid Crisis

All sides of the political spectrum agree: America is in the midst of an opioid epidemic. There is explosion in the prescription and misuse of synthetic and nonsynthetic opiates to treat chronic pain. Centers for Disease Control and Prevention (2016) data show a three-fold increase in deaths due to opioids over the past ten years. The Substance Abuse and Mental Health Services Administration (SAMHSA) has joined several other American health agencies to prioritize services for opioid use. They recognized stigma as being one of the major barriers for engagement in these services. Recently, I was contacted by a Midwest office responsible for developing and implementing plans to address this stigma. They were asking for advice on how to decrease stigma in order to engage people with opioid-related health challenges in treatment. My experience illustrated two hurdles in addressing stigma of substance use disorder including opioid misuse.

1. How to do it? Public health advocates have a simple request; tell us how to stop the stigma. However, just as there is significantly less research that explains the stigma of substance use disorders, so research on how to fix these stigmas is absent. The advocate's task is to adapt recommendations about stigma change provided later in this book to the needs of people harmed by the stigma of substance use disorder. This significantly slows the emergent need for change in this health crisis.

2. How does stigma differ within the group of people with substance use disorders? Recently completed research by our group suggests the stigma of substance use disorders includes stereotypes of criminality and immorality; that, for example, "addicts" choose their addiction because they are amoral, which will likely lead to criminal behavior (Nieweglowski et al., 2017). Research needs to determine whether this kind of moral view of substance use disorder extends to people who seemed to have started their addiction as a result of unintended consequences from pain management.

REMOVING PUBLIC STIGMA

Social psychological research on ethnic minority and other group stereo-types provides important insight on the effectiveness of strategies for reducing mental illness stigma of the public type. Based on this literature, I have grouped various approaches to changing public stigma into three processes: protest, education, and contact. These are summarized in table 2.2, briefly reviewed here, and then the mainstay of subsequent chapters of the book. *Protest* highlights injustices of various forms of stigma and chastises stigmatizers for their prejudice and discrimination. Disrespectful headlines might be used in protest programs to decrease stigma. People are then aware that these are unacceptable views about mental health which need to be stopped. Anecdotal evidence suggests that protest can have impact on some *behaviors*. For example, media groups may retract stigmatizing efforts in response to concerted efforts of advocates. But research also suggests protest can lead to attitude rebound effects.

TABLE 2.2 PROCESSES BY VEHICLES TO MAKE SENSE OF HOW TO CONFRONT STIGMA

	PROCESS		
VEHICLES	PROTEST	EDUCATION	CONTACT
Media-based	PSAs against movies like *Psycho*.	Video that reviews myths and facts.	Magazine story about individuals who tell peers about their experiences with mental illness.
In Vivo	A group that gathers in front of a movie theater against *Psycho*.	Psychiatrists at a community meeting who answer questions about mental illness and effective treatments.	Individuals with mental illness who tell their stories of mental illness at a community gathering.

Note: PSA is public service announcement.

"Don't tell me what to think. I'll believe people with mental illness are fundamentally incompetent if I want to."

Educational approaches to stigma change challenge inaccurate stereotypes about mental illness and replace these stereotypes with factual information.

> MYTH: People with serious mental illness will never recover, instead living out their lives on the back ward of a psych hospital.
> FACT: Recovery is the rule, not the exception.

Educational strategies aimed at reducing mental illness stigma have used public service announcements, books, flyers, movies, videos, and other audio visual aids to dispel myths about mental illness and replace them with facts. Educational approaches are especially popular as efficient ways to right social injustices.

The third strategy for reducing stigma is interpersonal *contact* with members of the stigmatized group. People from the general public who meet those with mental illness in recovery will significantly change their stigmatizing attitudes and behaviors. Contact's benefits are enhanced when it is with a person who moderately disconfirms the stereotypes about his or her group. Individuals who highly disconfirm prevailing stereotypes may not be believed as representative, instead being viewed as "special exceptions." Meeting famous people like movie stars or politicians with mental illness is less effective than interacting with the "average" person, the individual we sit next to every day at the office or share a pew with at church. Contact with persons who behave in ways consistent with the stereotypes about their group may reinforce stigmatizing attitudes or make them worse. Hence, meeting a person who is obviously psychotic—who is shouting aloud to her voices on the street—does not lessen stigma. Research has also defined what makes for a good recovery story, one that will diminish stigma. They include on-the-way-down stories where people share symptoms and disabilities that challenge them. On-the-way-down stories are necessary for the public to believe the person they are meeting, who looks so competent, actually had experiences that put them in the serious mental illness group. This is balanced with on-the-way up stories, experiences with personal achievements and hope. On-the-way-up stories embody recovery and eat away at the public's stigmatizing predilections.

VEHICLES FOR STIGMA CHANGE

What are the vehicles for protest, education, and contact to actually be shepherded into the real world? Table 2.2 distinguishes two: media-based strategies and in vivo or face-to-face approaches. Vehicles of both types are most effective when they are targeted. While changing an entire population's attitudes and behavior toward a stigmatized group is laudatory, history has rarely found it to occur. Instead, anti-stigma programs need to be targeted with the target being people who by virtue of their role are in positions of power vis-à-vis the stigmatized group. This would include employers for people with mental illness seeking a vocation, landlords for those wanting comfortable housing, health care providers for those seeking health and wellness, and faith leaders for those seeking acceptance into their communities. Targets might include noncommissioned officers for those seeking military careers, legislators when growing mental health programs are needed, and police for those engaged in the criminal justice system. Targets define the message, the recovery narrative that is likely to sway opinions of these groups. Employers, for example, are told that people with mental illness are capable of completing jobs competently, especially when they can avail themselves of reasonable accommodations. Targets also defined change goals. Stigma programs targeting employers are successful when people with mental illness are being hired and provided accommodations in the breadth and depth of the work world.

MEDIA-BASED APPROACHES

Public service announcements (PSAs) embedded in social-marketing campaigns are the best example of media effects. Social marketing is a collection of principles and practices meant to move forward an agenda reflecting social justice and health promotion. Social marketing is the umbrella program that integrates education and contact strategies meant to introduce and maintain change effects. These materials often include paper and online resources where interested viewers can learn more about mental illnesses and treatment of these disorders. First for most of these kinds of campaigns is the PSA, which is meant to activate and orient targeted viewers to public service campaign materials. PSAs are defined here as short audio and/ or video spots that have mostly been disseminated to television and radio networks, though they have recently spread to Internet social networking sites like Facebook, Pinterest, Instagram, and LinkedIn. Blogs and twitters may be additional innovative venues for PSAs.

Major anti-stigma campaigns and their PSAs have been developed and undertaken in the United Kingdom, Australia, Canada, United States, and other Western countries. Americans seem to have first developed formal media campaigns against stigma after the 1999 White House Conference on Mental Health. Tipper Gore and Alma Powell formed the National Mental Health Awareness Campaign. Among its materials were PSAs featuring adolescents forthrightly discussing their experiences with serious mental illness. They especially distributed the PSAs to teen-friendly media like MTV. Since then, the SAMHSA has been a national leader in anti-stigma efforts. They developed the ADS Center (Resource Center to Promote Acceptance, Dignity and Social Inclusion Associated with Mental Health). On the website is the Campaign for Mental Health Recovery produced by SAMHSA in partnership with the Ad Council. The campaign was partly informed by findings from President George W. Bush's New Freedom Commission.

IN VIVO APPROACHES TO CHANGING PUBLIC STIGMA

Perhaps the greatest benefit of media campaigns is breadth of impact; televised and online anti-stigma strategies have the broadest impact on stigma, helping the message get out to the "normal" majority. In vivo approaches offer a different perspective. Proponents of this strategy believe better effects occur when the targeted group is able to interact with people in recovery, where the interaction gives a chance for a free exchange of ideas about the person's experiences. This exchange provides for a veritable "test" of one's stereotypes. Members of the targeted group can check out for themselves whether the "mentally ill" person shows evidence of their stigmatizing view.

A target can discern in a one-to-one exchange whether the labeled person is unpredictable, incompetent, or dangerous. People with lived experience in much of the Western world have organized into speakers' bureaus with members ready to tell their recovery stories in formats relevant for different targets. Speakers' bureaus, for example, might be commissioned to speak to civic groups such as Rotary, collections of business leaders who are in positions to employ or rent to those with mental illness.

IMPACTING SELF-STIGMA

There are two broad approaches for replacing self-stigma with personal empowerment that somewhat parallel the education and contact distinctions of public stigma change. First, people might overcome self-stigma when they learn to challenge the myths of mental illness with facts. This process is more effective when individuals learn cognitive therapy strategies to challenge idiosyncratic ways in which people internalize stereotypes. Second, people are better able to deal with stigma through peer support. This effort requires decisions about disclosing one's mental health experiences.

EDUCATION AND COGNITIVE THERAPY

One promising approach is the "Ending Self-Stigma" (ESS) intervention, which uses a group approach to reduce self-stigmatization (Lucksted et al., 2011). ESS participants meet as a group for nine sessions with materials covering education about mental health, cognitive behavioral strategies to impact the internalization of public stigmas, methods to strengthen family and community ties, and techniques for responding to public discrimination. The cognitive behavioral strategies frame self-stigma as *irrational* self-statements (for example, "I must be a stupid person because I get depressed.") that the person seeks to challenge ("Most other people do not think depressed people are stupid."). These kinds of challenges lead to counters—pithy statements people might use next time they catch themselves self-stigmatizing. "There I go again. Just because I got depressed last fall does not mean I am stupid and incapable of handling a job. I have struggles just like everyone else."

PEER SUPPORT AND DISCLOSURE

Peer support programs offer another way for people with serious mental illness to enhance their sense of empowerment. Groups like these provide a range of services including support for those who are just coming out, recreation and shared experiences that foster a sense of community within a larger hostile culture, and advocacy/political efforts to further promote group pride. Several forces have converged over the past century to foster consumer-operated services for persons with psychiatric disabilities. Some reflect dissatisfaction with mental health services that disempower persons by providing services in restrictive settings. Others represent a natural tendency of persons to seek support from others with similar problems. Recently, a variety of peer-operated service programs have developed including: drop-in centers, housing programs, homeless services, case management, crisis response, benefit acquisition, anti-stigma services, advocacy, research, technical assistance, and employment programs.

Taking advantage of peer support requires coming out; to let other people know about the person's psychiatric history. "Coming out of the closet" with mental illness is associated with decreased self-stigmatization and improved quality of life. When people are open about their condition, worry and concern over secrecy is reduced, they may soon find peers or family members who will support them even after knowing their condition, and they may find that their openness promotes a sense of power and control over their lives. Still, being open about one's condition has its risks. Openness may bring about discrimination by members of the public, any relapses may be more widely known than preferred and therefore more stressful, and in some cases, disclosure may be more isolating. For example, in India, documentation of mental illness is grounds for divorce, a situation that some would consider a form of institutionalized stigma. A person with mental illness in India may feel doubly stressed by the threat of divorce and further public discrimination. Deciding to disclose is ultimately a very personal decision, closely tied to the cultural context, and requires thorough consideration of the potential benefits and consequences.

Coming out is not a black-or-white decision. There are strategies that vary in risk for handling disclosure. At the most extreme, people may stay in the closet through social avoidance. This means keeping away from situations where people may find out about one's mental illness. Instead, they only associate with other persons who have mental illness. It is protective (no one will find out the shame) but obviously also very restrictive. Others may choose not to avoid social situations but instead to keep their experiences a secret. An alternative version of this is selective disclosure. Selective disclosure means there is a group of people with whom private information is disclosed and a group from whom this information is kept secret. While there may be benefits of selective disclosure such as an increase in supportive peers, there is still a secret that could represent a source of shame. People who choose indiscriminant disclosure abandon the secrecy. They make no active efforts to try to conceal their mental health history and experiences. Hence, they opt to disregard any of the negative consequences of people finding out about their mental illness. Broadcasting one's experience means educating people about mental illness. The goal here is to seek out people to share past history and current experiences with mental illness. Broadcasting has additional benefits compared to indiscriminant disclosure. Namely, it fosters their sense of power over the experience of mental illness and stigma.

WHO IS HARMED BY THE STIGMA OF MENTAL ILLNESS?

Everyone is challenged by mental illness; everyone remembers times of depression or sadness in their life. We are all stressed by demands of growing up and becoming independent, establishing ourselves in careers, and building a family. We all know the depression of loss, death of loved ones, or failure to meet personal goals. The difference is that some of us are disabled by the experience. These momentary challenges of mental illness seem to extend and derail pursuit of aspirations. Some of us are marked by these

My coming out is an ever-evolving journey. I spent the first fifteen years of my professional career on faculty of two medical schools. I was in a culture where taking responsibility for the "mentally ill"—making wise treatment decisions in their absence of insight—was top priority, a culture I accepted, at the time. Our priority was to protect people from their mental illness by hook or by crook. Although wounded healers are common metaphors for mental health professionals, I was aware colleagues look askance at the psychologist who could not manage his illness. I also knew about the gallows humor that punctuates our practice. Some professionals might laugh off those overwhelmed by the troubles of our clients: "that's just a case of nuts running the nut house." Colleagues who were out with their mental illness were butts of these kinds of jokes. I continue today to hesitate coming out in grand rounds lectures to medical colleagues. I no longer care about their disapproval of me, only that they might discount my science. "Corrigan's research is not rigorous because he is biased."

Despite this concern, I never really saw being in the closet as a mark of shame or something I needed to carefully guard. In part, the support of my wife combated this problem. And a noticeable change occurred when I did start to disclose my story to the public at large. I felt fuller, like the world is seeing me now, warts and all. I liked the complete "ME" being out there. Still, at times, I am concerned that disclosure is self-serving. Sometimes it seems that the net of mental illness and recovery includes everyone. Depression and anxiety are not rare; almost everyone has stories of overwhelming sadness, stress, and exhaustion. They handle it quietly and with dignity, seemingly not needing to be on a platform to tell their story. I come from a stoic family where public displays were not encouraged; as a child, my parents never discussed with relatives how my brother, Mike, and I were doing in school, even though Mike was the first to go to and successfully graduate from college. Perhaps my public disclosures are self-congratulatory pats on the back. I also have a more complex concern; I don't belong in the cadre of heroes that are out.

"I am not as sick as those who I admire." I never heard voices, never attempted suicide, and was only hospitalized once. I have not earned the right to step out with those who have had greater challenges.

I also loathe pity, absolutely hate it. I therefore do not want to tell my story if people sympathize with me. I remember in a men's group at church once telling my story when Bob clapped me on the shoulder and said, "Wow, Pat. You really deal with a lot. I'm impressed with everything you have done. People like you are really something!" I was ashamed and I was angry. "I didn't tell you this, Bob, so you would pity me." And I denied—"Not me Bob. I'm not like those people."—in the process sadly adding to public stigma.

Despite this, I now broadly and proudly share my mental health experiences when I speak about the harmful effects of stigma and the promotion of affirming attitudes such as recovery and empowerment. My story changes based on the audience and it evolves over time based on insights and concerns. But I remain confident that disclosure is the secret to elimination of both public and self-stigma, the sentinel point of this book developed fully in later chapters.

experiences as a result, and mental illness becomes part of our identity. This may occur because of symptoms and disabilities themselves, corresponding treatments, or subsequent reactions of others. Mental illness is added to the list of descriptors that make up one's identity in the here and now. "I am a husband, father, son, college graduate, psychologist, cancer survivor, and person with serious mental illness." Identity with mental illness becomes master status for some, rising to the top of self-statements; "My mental illness is the dominant aspect of my identity."

When practicing as a psychologist, I worked with people who were depressed and anxious. Through cognitive behavior therapy, we successfully tackled symptoms leading to remission, thereby closing the book on this life adventure. They go on with life forgetting about these episodes like someone might forget a bad winter flu. They are relatively unscathed by stigma because they do not perceive themselves in the group of "mentally ill" people. For others, the book remains open for a substantial amount of time, changing fundamental perceptions of who the person is. I have struggled with symptoms, treatments, and people's reactions for more than forty years; it is part of my identity. People who identify with mental illness are more likely to be victimized by its stigma. They are also the group who fill the ranks of advocates and leaders of anti-stigma programs.

People who identify as advocates with lived experience often organize into communities with distinct agenda. There are people with lived experience, family members, providers, and interested parties organized into advocacy groups that specifically address mental illness or substance use disorder. Even within a broad class such as mental illness, I have worked with communities focusing on fetal alcohol spectrum disorder, suicide, Tourette's syndrome, and posttraumatic stress disorder. The communities comprise individuals who are energized and committed to erasing the stigma experienced by their community. Hence, experts working with them need to understand the collection of advocates has a history through which its perspectives on stigma and health developed. Experts need to respect this history. About five years ago I began to work with the community of Americans concerned about suicide stigma. As a clinical psychologist some twenty-five years ago, I learned suicide to be the result of mental illness and that killing one's self is "committing suicide." From advocates in this community, I learned viewing suicide through a mental illness lens limits understanding the entire experience and that "committing suicide" blames the person and is disrespectful. The community prefers "die by suicide." My work in this area required me to learn its history.

UNINTENDED CONSEQUENCES

This chapter lists the strategies on which progressives rely to tear down the stigma of mental illness. As written in the book's preface, progressives, by nature, want to be active using whatever insights exist from the rationale times in which we live to squash stigma and discrimination. In the process, we make mistakes. Social scientists have a name for this, the dodo bird effect.

Scientists want to progress but can be hampered by the dodo bird, a character from *Alice in Wonderland*. After judging a race among wonderlanders, dodo concludes, "Everybody has one and all must have prizes." Social scientist Saul Rosenzweig in 1936 used dodo's statement to reflect the state of research in behavior change; if everything works, then we don't know what to do. Consider the unlikely bedfellows of Freud's psychoanalysis and Skinner's behavior therapies. Original meta-analyses conducted by Lester Luborsky and colleagues in 1975 failed to show one approach outperforming another. This has several harmful effects. First, teachers and their students do not know what to learn and how to help. Is psychoanalysis as effective for depression as behavioral therapy? If I pick the wrong one, my client can suffer significant harm, perhaps even suicide. Second, policy makers do not know what interventions to promote. Third, lack of apparent distinctions can lead to unintended consequences. So if psychoanalysis works as well as behavior therapy, then therapists should adopt it for helping people with schizophrenia. Yet research since Luborsky and colleagues' 1970s analyses shows psychoanalysis not only to be feckless but to actually lead to harmful results. Some find the lack of direction and free associations of psychoanalysis overwhelming.

Stigma research has exploded in the past decades from only about sixty in the 1970s to more than 4500 since 2010. Hence, we benefit from a huge body of research to guide decisions about replacing stigma with affirming attitudes and behaviors. But we need to be mindful of the dodo bird effect to carefully identify well-intentioned approaches that not only fail to have meaningful effect but might actually worsen the status quo.

HOW TO EVALUATE ANTI-STIGMA PROGRAMS?

Readers, therefore, need to be mindful of how to rigorously study stigma, especially how to use valid methods and design to evaluate anti-stigma programs in terms of benefits and unintended harm. This is a complex enterprise with social scientists sifting through considerations of internal and external validity, psychometrics, randomized designs, and other aspects of esoterica; interested readers might wish to begin with a paper I authored with Jenessa Shapiro in 2010.

The lay reader should prioritize studies that reflect community-based participatory research (CBPR) embedded in the communities described earlier. Understanding stigma in terms of social justice and power calls for grassroots involvement in all aspects of science. Dissatisfaction with the status quo is typically championed by consumers of mental health services; hence, they need to be included in decisions about stigma programs, which means they need to have active roles in evaluations meant to inform these decisions. CBPR is the research agenda that includes people with lived experience as full partners with researchers in evaluation research. CBPR rests on two principles: perspective and politic. First, the backgrounds and varied perspectives inherent in CBPR partners with lived experience infuse theoretical understanding and corresponding research design with this diversity. Second, advocates flex their political power by consuming research findings, integrating them into policy, and using their authority and networks to realize important change.

What then does the CBPR team do? Similar to administrative councils of any human service program, the CBPR team is responsible for all activities related to research on stigma change programs that are then used to broaden campaigns meant to control prejudice and discrimination. This approach signals a paradigm shift for many researchers. Basic to CBPR, social scientists need to engage those with lived experience in effective evaluation. This includes understanding stigma problems, describing corresponding anti-stigma approaches, delineating methods and measures meant to test approaches, collecting and analyzing data that emerge from the design, and making sense of findings. Indeed, engagement is not sufficient as a descriptor. Partnership is more appropriate; scientists and people with lived experience share all decisions about a study. This means researchers need to educate stakeholders about key aspects of the research approach. However, CBPR is not unidirectional. People with lived experience, in turn, are responsible for educating researchers about the social significance of the goals of the study.

EFFECTS OF THE PROGRAM

The ultimate goal of stigma strategies is to lead to change in the real world, a considerable task when thinking about the breadth and depth of stigma in this thing called the *world*. Two concerns influence research when measuring these program effects especially as social marketing campaigns: penetration and impact. These concerns are also fundamental to marketing and might be understood in terms of increasing sales of a new product, for example, a dancing Coke can. Penetration is the extent to which the population remembers seeing the focus of the (social) marketing campaign: Coke or anti-stigma messages. What percent of a representative sample remembers seeing the dancing can in various media channels? Or how many in a group recall an anti-stigma education campaign? Impact represents the direct effect of the campaign. Coca-Cola wants to know whether people are buying more Coke as a result of the dancing can. Similarly, anti-stigma campaigns are effective to the degree they address the advocate's imperative. In the next chapter, I review three agendas that embody the central goals of anti-stigma programs.

3

THREE COMPETING AGENDAS
TO ERASE STIGMA

B EATING STIGMA SEEMS obvious—Stop it!—but to what end? Some
advocates believe stigma dissuades people from seeking out services
when needed because of label avoidance. Erasing this kind of stigma
removes barriers to getting help. Some believe discrimination against
people with mental illness robs them of rightful opportunities, the egregious effect of public stigma. Erasing public stigma erases hurdles to
achieving personal goals in education, employment, independent living,
relationships, and health. Some believe self-stigma leads to shame, forcing
people into the closet to keep their experiences secret. Addressing self-
stigma helps people out of the dark, replacing feelings of shame with those
of pride and self-esteem. Hence, there are three different agendas that
define anti-stigma programs:

- *The SERVICES Agenda*, decrease label avoidance so people engage in
  evidence-based services.
- *The RIGHTS Agenda*, decrease public stigma so people enjoy rightful life
  opportunities.
- *The SELF-WORTH Agenda*, decrease self-stigma to replace shame with
  dignity.

The trouble is that agendas sometimes compete or conflict with each
other. The stigma effect blinds us to the difference. Advocates, in their zeal

to correct "stigma," are unaware that specific agendas may differ and that attempting to resolve one problem might actually worsen another. In this chapter, I show how agendas are fairly specific in effects, improving service seeking, for example, but having no impact on rights or self-worth. Even more, efforts to promote one agenda might worsen another; for example, some attempts to promote services through stigma elimination might reduce rights. Hence, being mindful of differing agendas is an essential first step in crafting anti-stigma efforts.

THE SERVICES AGENDA: HELPING PEOPLE INTO EVIDENCE-BASED CARE

In chapter 2, I defined label avoidance as a type of stigma that causes major barriers to seeking treatment services. Although there are several evidence-based practices for people with serious mental illness, many individuals opt not to seek these services in time of need or drop out of them prematurely (SAMHSA, 2013). This occurs because people want to avoid providers and places where users are associated with stigmatizing labels. The Services Agenda seeks to replace label avoidance with a certain sense of optimism so that people are more willing to engage in care. One way Services Agendas do this is by promoting mental health literacy through social marketing and communication campaigns. Anthony Jorm, a world leader in literacy from Australia, defines mental health literacy as education about mental illness, which aids in recognition, management, and prevention. Typically, first in literacy campaigns are succinct statements about specific mental illnesses—depression, anxiety, schizophrenia—as "treatable disorders like most physical illnesses." As there is no shame in having cancer or heart disease, individuals who better recognize their mental illness and corresponding treatment options better avail those options.

An Australian program called *beyondblue* has a long history of pursuing the Services Agenda. *beyondblue* is a social marketing campaign that includes public service announcements (PSAs) framing *depression* as a treatable disease. The focus of *beyondblue* has evolved its audience priorities over time. For example, *beyondblue* has been concerned about men and mental health in the past few years because men are less likely to admit to mental health challenges or engage in treatment. As a result, they launched Man Therapy that included humorous ways to entice men into mental health care.

> Blokes. They're happy to get all touchy-feely on the sporting field, but when it comes to getting in touch with their feelings and emotions, on the 'NOT' sporting field, sometimes known as 'life', they tend to drop the ball. So the shit hits the fan and that's a mess nobody in their right mind wants to clean up, believe me.
>
> Well men, it's time to pick up your game and grab the bull by the horns. Better yet, grab the bull by the balls! That's if it'll let you. And bloody well get on with it! Hello, I'm Doctor Brian Ironwood. Go ahead, have a rummage around my site. You might just learn something about yourself, like how much you love grilled pineapple.
>
> (retrieved from https://www.mantherapy.org.au/ December 21, 2016)

Doctor Ironwood's site includes buttons on Man Facts, Man Therapies, and Tales of Triumph. It also includes hotline numbers and strategies for immediate emergency support. *beyondblue* has been active in Australia for almost fifteen years and shown to have penetrated the population well with 60 percent of Australians aware of the program (Highet, Luscombe, Davenport, Burns, & Hickie, 2006). Campaign awareness was associated with better recognition of mental illnesses and greater understanding of treatment benefits (Jorm, Christensen, & Griffiths, 2005).

Mental Health First Aid (MHFA) is another mental health literacy program, originating in Australia and expanding greatly across the United States and Canada during the past few years. MHFA is an eight-hour course taught in classroom settings that reviews basic information and skills so course participants can help others with mental health problems or crises. MHFA also has fairly vast penetration having been completed by more than 1 percent of Australians (Jorm & Kitchener, 2011). It was the centerpiece of U.S. legislation meant to address gun violence after Sandy Hook related to mental illness (HR 5996) with the ambitious intent to be presented to all of America's high school youth. Findings from a meta-analysis showed people who completed training were likely to have mastered information about mental illness and show diminished stigma (Hadlacsky, Hokby,

Mkrtchian, Carli, & Wasserman, 2014). This kind of information is expected to boost care seeking.

A Services Agenda focusing on mental health literacy can be assessed with obvious indicators of success. Evidence that people are more engaged in mental health care after anti-stigma programs demonstrates benefits of a Services Agenda. Care seeking, however, is a complex construct, partly moderated by label avoidance but also influenced by additional social determinants. These include availability and accessibility. Have mental health systems and local governments invested in evidence-based programs so they are available to interested parties without long wait times or excessive cost? Are available services also accessible? In cities, this means, can they be reached by public transportation in areas relatively free from concerns of crime? Accessibility is even more challenging in rural settings where tens to hundreds of miles separate people from evidence-based programs. Cultural relevance is a third determinant of service use. At a minimum, are services provided to people in their first language and not limited to English? Mexicans living in the United States for less than a year are unlikely to benefit from mental health services unless they are provided in Spanish. Even more, are interventions relevant to the ethnic or religious group of people who might seek services? Evidence-based practices in the United States typically represent Western priorities of individualism where decision making is driven by the patient. These may seem foreign to collectivist cultures that, for example, may prefer to have families actively involved in services.

What advocates are likely to endorse a Services Agenda? They are people confident that existing evidence-based services can meaningfully help those in need of mental health care. Prominent among these are mental health professionals: psychiatrists, psychologists, and others with graduate-level training. They know from firsthand experience the beneficial effects of services they provide. Health professional agendas are often echoed by community leaders. Getting people into treatment, for example, is frequently endorsed by legislators when making funding decisions. Professionals and community leaders are joined by large systems, e.g., wraparound collections of inpatient and outpatient mental health programs targeting diverse arrays of illnesses for people of varied ages. Pharmaceutical companies are also prominent in a Services Agenda. This partly represents their genuine concern about patient populations. But it may also reflect efforts to expand markets thereby growing product sales. In the latter case, concerns arise about whether a Services Agenda represents interest of patient or profit.

Family members often endorse a Services Agenda. Parents, in particular, are concerned about children with mental illness who are not benefiting from evidence-based care. This concern can escalate to legitimate worry about adult children ending up homeless, victims of crime, or snared by the criminal justice system. Earlier, I noted that the family agenda is not synonymous with people with lived experience. Families worried about their loved ones are enamored by potential benefits of evidence-based strategies, sometimes overlooking their harmful side effects in the process. Families might prefer interventions that urge caution toward relapse. People with lived experience who have suffered side effects might be less drawn to such treatments in the future. People with lived experience might tire of caution, instead preferring strategies that get them back in the job market or living independently quicker.

Despite these concerns, there are still many individuals with mental illness who endorse a Services Agenda. They are people who have previously enjoyed the successes of evidence-based interventions. Their stories of recovery that resulted from treatment are especially compelling elements of effective campaigns meant to impact the Services Agenda.

THE RIGHTS AGENDA: REPLACING DISCRIMINATION WITH AFFIRMING ATTITUDES AND BEHAVIORS

Public stigma robs people of rights to a complete education, good jobs, nice place to live, satisfactory health care, and intimate relationships. A Rights Agenda mirrors civil rights movements of the past fifty years seeking to advance opportunities and quality of life for people of color, women, and the lesbian, gay, bisexual, transgender, questioning (LGBTQ) community. The Rights Agenda embodies social injustice concerns of mental illness stigma. It mobilizes the rectitude of intent that represents civil rights movements around the world by appealing to the progressives' sense of right and wrong. The clarion call to righteousness empowers messaging, giving them an assertive quality not seen in the "sales" approach of Services Agendas.

I am a licensed clinical psychologist with more than twenty-five years of experience focused on symptoms and disabilities of people with serious mental illnesses including schizophrenia and bipolar disorder. The first half of my career was spent at the University of Chicago Medical School as director of what was called at the time an "aftercare program" for people with serious mental illness— services for people after they were discharged from inpatient psychiatric hospitalization. We were a community-based program in six cottages on the grounds of Tinley Park Mental Health Center, a state hospital in the southwest suburbs of Chicago.

I was convinced that our evidence-based approaches helped those who engaged in them. Therefore, I was frustrated by those who chose not to use our program. I felt at the time that they were misguided about benefits of these interventions and that, sometimes, their decisions went astray because of diminished insight due to the illness. In chapter 1, I unpacked the misassumptions of nonadherence, replacing the idea in later years with insights on self-determination. Back then I pursued strategies that motivated participants to engage in our treatments. That is why I endorsed the Services Agenda when I understood the harmful effects of label avoidance. Strategies that tear down stigma will reduce one of the biggest disincentives to care seeking and help people become more engaged.

Protest seems to be an especially appropriate approach to accomplishing the Rights Agenda. Organized programs that shout out disrespectful messages and demand opportunity for people with lived experience may be the first steps in efforts to regain rights. Rights programs have also included education and contact. Opening Minds is a nationwide effort in Canada that largely rests on contact-based interventions to address rights. Opening Minds sought to build networks of practice, collections of small, contact-based programs from across the country that were reimbursed for local anti-stigma-based efforts. Preliminary analyses may suggest that contact programs have positive effects on targeted groups of youth, health care providers, Canadians in the workplace, and the media (Stuart et al., 2014).

Although the Rights Agenda is a bit ethereal, resting on a pillar of justice, its goals are obvious and accountable. Evidence that people are benefiting from education opportunities with suitable supports, being hired and offered reasonable accommodations, finding comfortable living, enjoying intimate relationships, and enjoying solid health care shows a Rights Agenda is successful. Assertive demands of people with lived experience have also been used by proponents of a Services Agenda to help the "normal" majority understand that mental illness, and corresponding help, is not limited to the disrespected or downtrodden.

Progressives of all stripes are drawn to the Rights Agenda. Agenda leaders need to be more narrowly defined from this group because people with lived experience are the legitimate owners of anti-stigma programs. People of color need to lead the fight against racism, women against sexism, and LGBTQ community against homophobia. I am a white, straight, male, not from any of these communities, per se. I hugely endorse and do my best to promote them, but my legitimacy in leading them is lacking. Cases where sexism is addressed without having women front and center yield disempowering messages that undercut a woman's authority: "she needs a man to speak for her!" This does not mean I have no value in civil rights efforts. I do so, as an ally. Solidarity is the goal here; I stand *with* oppressed people, lending my voice and resources to further goals of social justice. But I do so from the backseat in a trip mapped by those who are harmed by stigma. Hence, my role in a Rights Agenda against mental illness stigma is very different when I am a person with lived experience versus a licensed clinical psychologist—driving in the former case, following in the latter.

Backseats can be unsettling for allies. Most human service providers, for example, entered the field drawn by compassion and desire to help people with health challenges. Mental health seems to be especially compelling because depression and anxiety are private experiences that tear up all of us. We are often called wounded healers to reflect the personal travails that lead us into the field. In addition, we are usually expected as providers to lead evidence-based interventions. Doctors are especially the ones in charge. Mental health providers were also among the first to point out the unfairness embodied in stigma. The World Psychiatric Association, for example, launched an international anti-stigma effort more than a decade ago. Being put in the backseat seems to ignore professional priorities as well as its power.

An equally ironic group of allies pushed to the backseat are family members. Parents often find their adult children with serious mental illness ill-served by community mental health systems. As a result, parents developed an assertive voice to assure loved ones got services and opportunities they were entitled to. In fact, in the 1960s the National Alliance on Mental Illness (NAMI) developed a coordinated advocacy effort representing concerns of families and their loved ones with mental health challenges. Families did this with the sincere belief that efforts were driven by the best interests of their relatives. In considering front and back seat, I do not believe families should cede advocacy roles. Many people with serious mental illness have been blessed by the commitment and energy of parents or older siblings, partnerships that are often essential for recovery. But most parents also realize that some form of recovery and self-determination is necessary during a person's journey to recovery. Parents speaking for the person with mental illness accentuates the belief that they are unable to speak for themselves and undermines self-determination. Hence, beating stigma experienced by the person with mental illness relegates parents to allies.

The picture gets a bit more complex, however, when considering family stigma—that, for example, mothers and fathers are to blame for the serious mental illness of their children and therefore need to be strategically distanced from them for the recovery process. Blame and disrespect are family stereotypes with families victimized by corresponding prejudice and discrimination. Neighbors exclude them from parties, bosses limit advancements, and landlords withhold leases, all because they are disdained for what they did to their child. In this case, family members drive a Rights Agenda. Family members must manage a delicate balancing act, making sure parents, for example, speak for themselves when addressing family stigma and not wander into anti-stigma assertions for their children.

Civil rights campaigns have amazing heroes that embody the movement: Martin Luther King Jr., and Mohandas Gandhi righting prejudice against people of color; Susan B. Anthony and Jane Addams promoting women's rights; and Harvey Milk championing gay agendas. Mental health has its heroes too. Clifford Beers, a Yale graduate, was hospitalized with psychosis in private and state hospitals of Connecticut from 1900 to 1903. This is more than a century ago. If we think people with mental illness generate public feelings of fear and confusion now, imagine what it was like during the age of asylums when people were shipped off to faraway institutions. Yet Beers believed efforts to improve mental health services begin assertively with those who have received these services: "I must fight in the open!" (Beers, 1909). Clifford Beers started the National Committee for Mental Hygiene, which since evolved into Mental Health America (MHA). MHA describes itself as "the nation's leading community nonprofit dedicated to helping Americans achieve wellness by living mentally healthier lives (http://www.mentalhealthamerica.net/who-we-are)." They accomplish their goals with members and affiliates in all fifty states.

THE SELF-WORTH AGENDA: REPLACING THE CLOSET WITH COMING OUT PROUD

The Self-Worth Agenda addresses harmful effects of self-stigma that lead to beliefs that people with mental illness should be ashamed of themselves. The Self-Worth Agenda strives to replace shame with feelings of pride. People with lived experiences themselves first recognized and challenged these beliefs. We Are Not Alone, a group of ex-patients in the 1940s from Rockland State Hospital gathered on the steps of the New York Public Library to offer mutual support. In the process, they learned that promoting personal empowerment was effective to erase self-stigma. Since then, thousands of mutual help and peer services have developed across the country, with Substance Abuse and Mental Health Services (SAMHSA) now supporting three national technical assistance centers with missions specific to this effort. As defined in chapter 2, mutual help and peer support programs are developed and operated by people with mental illness, for people with mental illness. They are often augmented by disclosure programs, those that help people decide about strategically disclosing their mental health experiences to promote empowerment.

The Self-Worth Agenda is led by people with lived experience, especially those who may have internalized stigma in their recovery. Ironically, those who might *benefit* from Self-Worth priorities may not be aware of its

One of the most chilling moments of my life occurred when calling my wife from the unit's wall phone asking her to explain to my children that "dad's in the hospital." And then twelve-year-old Liz coming that night with "deer in the headlight eyes" being in the psych unit. Dad among all these whacked out patients. Having a serious mental illness, dropping out of school, quitting jobs, getting hospitalized; what's to be proud of?

Despite my share of mental health challenges, I somehow got through school, earned a doctorate, and became a professor, rising to be one of the dozen distinguished professors at the university. All this occurred on the back of more than 350 peer-reviewed journal articles and fifteen books. I have reason to be proud. But, managing my disability is a far greater accomplishment. Being able to live, work, and love my family while at times being paralyzed by anxiety, overwhelmed by sadness, and preoccupied with death is an even greater accomplishment that I can achieve despite the challenges, and is worth celebrating. We must, however, be cautious about what is meant by achievement. Surpassing disability does not require becoming an Olympic sportsman or Nobel laureate or college professor. My dad was a sixty-hour-per-week electrical contractor for his working life. My mother was his bookkeeper until she was seventy-five. This is proud. My wife was a public defender for thirty years; pride. Yeomen should be celebrated.

But even here, accomplishment is not set by an external bar. Everyone can achieve with the definition of success set by their own agenda. Hence, the person who has been bedridden due to paralyzing depression has achieved when she is able to get to church three times a week for her volunteer job. The person who, despite significant social anxiety, is able to go to a movie with a friend has succeeded. The person, despite the voices of psychosis, who is able to finish adult education on local politics should celebrate.

Pride has a second element entwined with the idea of identity. Patrick Corrigan is an Irish name, and every March 17, I proudly celebrate Saint Paddy's day when Chicago dyes our river green. I

(continued)

do nothing to achieve this, but it's part of who I am. Expressing identity is welded to pride. Most people's identity is multileveled. I am a psychologist, a professor, a husband, a father, a father-in-law, a runner, a tinkerer. I am from Evanston Illinois, went to college in Omaha, and trained in southern California. And I am a person with mental illness. For some people, mental illness is part of their identity; *not* in the broken and recovered sense—I was depressed but now I am healed. Rather, the sum of challenges, treatments, reactions, and recovery define a large chunk of one's life adding to I-statements: "And I have a mental illness." Mental health experiences as part of authenticity is not a need for everyone. I have worked with people in my clinical practice, challenged by depression, who have benefited by therapy, closed the book on this experience, and gone on with their lives. But there are people like me, moved or marked by their experience, needing to share all aspects of their identity with pride.

importance. These are people who think shame is a natural consequence of mental illness and remain closeted and secret. Hence, one goal of the Self-Worth Agenda is to trumpet the importance of empowerment broadly so those hiding their experience might find peers who will support their journey to disclosure. We see this in other advocacy groups. Members of the LGBTQ community, for example, often organize with peers to gain support and energy in the pursuit of their efforts. Once again, allies are important here. One group in the gay community is Parents, Families, and Friends of Lesbians and Gays. In addition, NAMI members often assume ally roles to support advocates with lived experiences.

AGENDAS COMPETE

In the zeal to repudiate stigma, many believe all good-intentioned efforts are effective, an idea I seek to replace with the critical appraisals highlighted in this book. Not every approach to stigma change works equally, with some strategies actually making things worse. Distinguishing among the three agendas is useful for this critical enterprise. The three approaches differ in fundamental purposes, processes, and messages, which influence the lens through which specific strategies are analyzed. The Services Agenda, for example, seeks to destigmatize mental illnesses by framing them as treatable disorders, which can lead to unintended consequences for a Rights Agenda. Framing a person in terms of a treatable disease is meant to assuage concern about the efficacy of interventions. "Depression is an illness like high blood pressure; both are easily treatable." But stressing *treatable disease* accentuates the idea of difference, that the person with depression is somehow not like the "normal" majority. And people who are different are somehow broken. Difference in mental health, unlike in blood pressure, leads to disdain.

A focus on treatable disease may also turn narratives about mental illness and stigma to pity. Although pity and sympathy are driven by benevolent wishes of the "normal" majority, research by our group mostly shows untoward effects of pity (Fominaya, Corrigan, & Rüsch, 2016). Those with mental illness who pity peers are likely to view those peers with more stigma and as dangerous, leading to greater social avoidance. Pity also turns inward to troubling effects. People with lived experience who view their mental health experiences with pity show diminished self-esteem and powerlessness, which can ironically lead to greater depression! A pity message echoes old notions of charity where people of advantage *bestow* opportunities on the needy. This dated idea has been replaced by a mandate for empowerment. Everyone has a right to opportunity; those with advantage should make sure all have power to obtain these opportunities. I do not mean to say that "treatable disease" as an effort to decrease label avoidance and get people into care fails to have benefits, only that proponents of a services view need to be mindful of its unintended effects on Rights Agendas.

Advocates also need to be aware that the three agendas compete for limited resources. Summaries of government programs with five-to-ten-year histories in the United States, United Kingdom, Canada, and Australia show they are limited by available funds to stoke their budgets. As a result, choices need to be made between, for example, agendas by social marketing campaigns to enhance service seeking versus those for grassroots efforts to promote rights and self-worth. McCrone, Knapp, and colleagues (2010) offered a useful method for translating the cost-effectiveness of specific anti-stigma programs into ratios of costs per citizen in a geographic area and benefits such as change in population attitudes leading to better work or independent living. Metrics such as these can be used by policy makers to apportion monies accordingly.

Implementing agendas is also limited by the public's attention. Some psychologists understand attention and overall condition as a limited resource (Kahneman, 1973). A person can process only so much informa-tion over time. Most Westerners are bombarded by well-intentioned public service announcements meant to provide wisdom on a slew of worthy health priorities as well as social justice issues ad infinitum. In turn, this information stands alongside other media onslaught experienced by people each day. Hence, cognitive space for tackling stigma has its limits. As an overall plan, advocates need to discern how any one message serving an anti-stigma agenda cuts into the overall pie of anti-stigma goals, another focus of anti-stigma policy.

Well-intentioned advocates might seek to address limited cognitive resources by crafting anti-stigma programs like a smorgasbord, believing more desirable programs combine all sorts of strategies. Programs integrate education, contact, and protest with a variety of topics using multiple media options. They target the goals of all three agendas. Perhaps one of the ele-ments of such a hybrid approach will hit the mark like a shotgun blast. I know of a college toolkit that engages students in a four-year program of stigma change focusing on care seeking, rights, and service agendas. Does this kind of *mishegas* really yield meaningful change? One of the benefits of scientists in the anti-stigma effort is development of theory that guides what we know about stigma and stigma change. The smorgasbord fails to thoughtfully integrate theory into a meaningful package. As just demon-strated, pushing for mental illness as treatable disease in order to enhance care seeking may undermine the Rights Agenda. I do believe broad-based efforts to change stigma may have an advantage, but evidence is necessary to show that advocates thoughtfully weave together approaches and meth-ods instead of heaping all from the menu onto their tray.

Policy decisions like these must be kept in mind as we consider how agendas differ by power base. Services Agendas are eagerly endorsed by professional groups. Psychiatric and psychological associations are able to muster loud voices that focus public attention on label avoidance and care seeking. Pharmaceutical companies kick in funds to support this agenda. Families buttonhole legislators to support these goals. The power base behind goals of Rights and Self-Worth Agendas seem to pale in comparison. Traditionally, people with lived experience were dismissed as "patients" with less legitimacy. Fortunately, the personal power agenda of advocates with lived experience is growing in its influence over community and government priorities. This might be traced back in the United States to George W. Bush's New Freedom Commission of 2002 where the president purposefully integrated advocates with lived experience into the commission; they, in turn, made sure empowerment and recovery were prominent in the final report. Since then, state and local governments have placed people with lived experience on mental health committees with the power to make funding decisions about service and community programs including anti-stigma efforts. In some ways, this reflects the evolving wisdom of social justice efforts discussed previously in this book, that people who are victims of stigma, prejudice, and discrimination—people of color, with differing sexual orientation, or with mental illness—need to be leading efforts to erase this injustice.

WHOSE WAR IS IT?

The war against racism is led by people of color, against sexism by women, and against homophobia by the LGBTQ community. Efforts to erase the stigma of mental illness come from different quarters. Changes to the mental health system have traditionally been led by providers and administrators. They have knowledge of illness and intervention that help them evolve programs to be the most effective. They attacked stigma as a way to get patients more involved in care and government funders to more fully support them. Feeling left out, family members organized into an effective voice to augment system change. Family members believed they were better able to understand in-the-street needs of loved ones. They joined anti-stigma movements to broaden treatment and independent-living

In May 2017, I met with an ad hoc faculty/staff/student committee at a distinguished Southern university to inform their nascent campaign on mental illness stigma. They were a well-intentioned and studious group committed to grasping the three agendas in order to meet overall goals of their community. "How, for example, do we balance needs to engage stressed students in care with priorities of students who no longer wish to hide their mental health experiences?" All was good until committee members recounted tragedies of the past year, students who were overwhelmed by mental health challenges and died by suicide. The discussion flipped. The priority was clear: no suicide was tolerable. The Services Agenda became the sole focus of the discussion. If need be, committee members were willing to jeopardize individual rights to safeguard students from suicide.

Suicide is the atomic bomb of mental health. It is the single issue that trumps all among psychiatric services. Suicide is the tragic sign of failure—not the disaster of people who died by suicide per se but rather the failing of the health care system meant to serve them. Public health campaigns have emerged to tackle this singular concern. *Zero Suicide* was launched nationwide in 2017.

I unequivocally endorse zero suicide. My grandfather died by suicide the day after Christmas when I was still an infant. I have personally experienced a life not worth living, that I'm better off dead. I am grateful that family and providers around me heard my sadness and stepped in. My first job in mental health was as an operator on a crisis line in Omaha. Late on a Sunday night in 1974, a caller died by suicide with me on phone. I have had therapeutic relationships with two people who died by suicide. The one absolute law of counseling I teach my students is that suicidal statements in session must be probed and prevention plans crafted. In no way as a helper do I view suicide as a philosophical conundrum worth debating. It is the sad result of mental illness that must be interdicted.

The problem occurs when we use zero suicide as the rationale for only addressing the Services Agenda. Rights must be addressed too.

options to relatives with mental illness. They frequently prioritize services agenda. People with lived experiences are seemingly late to the effort. While they recognize the importance of diminishing stigma on care seeking, they tend to be most vocal about Rights and Self-Worth Agendas.

Stigma change by triumvirate is different than programs to erase racism, sexism, and homophobia. I am a huge advocate of rights for people of color, women, and LGBTQ. But as a white heterosexual male, my role is relegated to ally. Allies are important in the back seat taking orders from the stigmatized community moving forward. Allies, however, do not set agenda. This is a very different vision than what drives mental illness stigma programs. One of the tasks going forward is for different constituencies to rearrange themselves to better understand and promote the agendas of people harmed by stigma, people with lived experience.

DO NOT GET MIRED IN HEADY THEORY

Pages in this chapter were a bit esoteric, taking something as important as goals for actually changing stigma and reducing them to notions of differing agendas, competing resources, and limited capacity. If these explanations help, then there is benefit in the distinction. But I always hail back to the advocates' imperative; namely, benefits of these and other considerations in the book are evinced only when they lead to important reductions in prejudice and discrimination as well as enhancements in affirming attitudes and behaviors.

4

IT IS MUCH MORE THAN
CHANGING WORDS

N O DOUBT ABOUT it, language worsens stigma; use of the "N" word, or bitch, or fag flames anger and hatred toward people of color, women, or individuals with minority sexual orientations. We recognize the unacceptable harm of words so much that most people will not even spell out the word for which "N" stands. Referring to them as African Americans, and women, and gays is a good start to undermine the prejudice and discrimination heinous terms like these embody. Hence, some advocates have said replacing bad words that describe people with stigmatized conditions might be an effective step for decreasing their experiences with prejudice and discrimination. Several coordinated efforts have therefore used word change as a way to tackle stigma. I briefly review these in this chapter as well as what research says about it. I cannot quarrel with the intent. Clearly, I choose my words carefully; for example, in referring to people with lived experience, I put the person first and refer to their condition not as illness but as life events. But like all intentions, I think word-focused anti-stigma programs yield unintended consequences that challenge their overall worth. Perhaps the biggest, and the best, example of the stigma effect is framing stigma change as the "easy" task of just changing the words.

CHANGING WORDS

Bruce Link, who completed some of the defining work in this area while at Columbia University, equated the mark of mental illness stigma with label. People labeled crazy or nuts are disparaged. Nor does a label's harm improve with clinical terms; calling people schizophrenic, manic, or agoraphobic is similarly hurtful. Advocates in other fields have recognized and tried to resolve this risk. Leprosy is now called Hansen's disease, dementia is Alzheimer's disease, and mental retardation is intellectual disability. In fact, cultural distaste has added "MR," or even worse just "R," alongside the "N" word as unspeakable in the American vernacular; an act of Congress actually removed "MR" from the federal lexicon. More recently, mental health advocates have searched for alternative words to replace various mental illness diagnoses and their labels. Given the especially stigmatizing experiences of those labeled with schizophrenia, renaming it has been particularly discussed. A survey by the World Psychiatric Association and European Psychiatric Association showed more than seventy-five experts of psychopathology endorsed renaming schizophrenia (Maruta, Volpe, Gaebel, Matsumoto, & Iimori, 2014). A slew of alternatives have been mentioned. Consistent with the presumed benefits of proper names such as those that occurred when dementia became known as Alzheimer's disease, proposals for alternative names of schizophrenia include Bleuler's syndrome and Kraepelin's disease for the psychiatrists who were among the first to describe the disorder, or John Nash syndrome for the Nobel laureate with schizophrenia who became more famous after his biopic, *A Beautiful Mind* starring Russell Crowe. Alternatively, labels have sought to describe characteristic symptoms of schizophrenia and include dysfunctional thought disorder; disorganized thinking disorder; and conative, cognitive, and reality distortion (also known as CONCORD; yikes, will the "normal" majority be able to learn this acronym?). Based on the belief that framing mental illness as medical disorders will decrease stigma related to blame, proposed changes include brain disintegration disorder and social brain disorder. (See Maruta and colleagues (2013) for a full discussion of these changes.)

East Asian professional associations have been especially active in pursuing name changes (Sartorius et al., 2014). The Japanese Society of

Psychiatry and Neurology altered the old term for schizophrenia, *Seishin-Bunretsu-Byo*, which translates as "mind-split disease" and is viewed as disrespectful in the vernacular, to *Togo-Shitcho-Sho*, which means "integration disorder" and is believed to be less degrading. Other Asian countries have followed suit including Korea: *Jeongshin-bunyeol-byung* (split mind disorder) to *Johyun-byung* (attunement disorder) and Hong Kong: *Jing Shen Fen Lis* (splitting of the mind) to *Si Jue Shi Tiao* (dysfunction of thought and perception). Researchers have used these changes to examine its effects on the "normal" majority as well as on mental health service providers. Although findings are complex, disparate conclusions emerge. The "normal" majority continues to be confused. To paraphrase, "It doesn't matter. Call them schizophrenic, Bleuler's disease, or brain disintegration disorder. They're still nuts!" Impact seems to be greater on providers with noticeable recognition and use of the name change. I doubt, however, that this represents a lessening of stigma as much as a *Diagnostic and Statistical Manual* (DSM) of the American Psychiatric Association effect. The DSM is the compendium of scientifically defined psychiatric syndromes, with its fifth edition (the DSM-5) in 2013. Most clinicians, me included, learn new labels quickly if we want to bill insurance companies appropriately or use correct terms in the professional journals. For example, Asperger's syndrome, a more benign form of autism, was removed from the DSM-5, instead embedding the concept in the broader term of Autism Spectrum Disorder. It has fallen from clinical discourse as a result. Service providers learn new terms for mental illnesses when formalized in the DSM for practice survival.

Let me be clear—words matter! I choose my words carefully and do not want to insult advocacy communities with whom I partner by using terms abhorrent to them. However, I think discussion about changing words is mostly talking to the choir. Progressives who already endorse ideas of recovery and self-determination will promote more-sensitive language. But this is a nuanced issue that will escape the "normal" majority who do not understand stigma. Those who continue to believe mental illness leads to unpredictable homicide are not going to be swayed by replacing schizophrenia with Bleuler's syndrome.

Notable strides in language have occurred in my lifetime progressing from the "N" word, to colored, to black, to African Americans. However,

I try to be attentive to words when publicly lecturing on the topic. I was keynoting a NAMI-California conference in Newport Beach in August 2015, trying to integrate an evolving interest in the stigma of mental health and substance use disorders. Substance Abuse and Mental Health Services (SAMHSA) likes to refer to these jointly as behavioral health, the term I used in Newport Beach. I talked about the stigma of behavioral health in order to avoid disrespecting anyone in the audience. During the Q&A, audience members hit me with two critiques about "behavioral health." One said he objected to the word *behavior* because it suggested people "chose" to be that way, that it's a behavior and not a medical condition with genetic origins. A second said she did not like grouping mental illness with substance use disorder under a single rubric suggesting, perhaps, that those with mental illness are tainted by association with those with more egregious (and more stigmatized) disorders.

I also tried to avoid word sins in my reference to mental illness. Many advocates with lived experience do not like illness as focus, medicalizing the issue with all the harm it evokes. In this spirit, I used mental health "challenge" in my NAMI speech. After, a person cornered me saying,

> "Mental health 'challenge!' What's that? I have a mental illness. 'Challenge' waters down the whole thing. Call it what it is: mental ILLNESS." The more I speak publicly about mental illness, the less certain I am about appropriate language.

just because we learned to change the words does not mean we eradicated prejudice and discrimination against people of color. David Sears (1988) was among the first to recast ethnic discrimination in America to what he called symbolic racism. The harsh laws of Jim Crow have disappeared, to be sure, but blacks are still victims of discrimination in work, housing, and health care settings. Racists have learned to pursue their agenda undercover. Effects of social desirability is one reason; people have learned that bigoted behavior is less tolerated in the modern world. Hence, people might still discriminate against blacks but do so while no longer using the "N" word.

Similarly, people might stop saying "schizo" but still choose not to hire individuals with mental illness.

WHAT SAYS THE CONSENSUS?

There is equal disagreement about what to call the focus of this book, people with the lived condition.

> He has schizophrenia. No, the person should never be limited by a diagnosis.
> She has a mental illness. No, descriptions should not be limited to the negative: illness.
> I have behavioral health challenges. No, I don't want to be lumped in with addicts.

Consensus would seem to be an empirical way to resolve the disagreement—what do people with lived experience agree is the way to refer to this experience? Research, however, fails to find agreement about best words (Mueser, Glynn, Corrigan, & Baber, 1996; Penn & Nowlin-Drummond, 2001). One decades-old argument examined in public surveys was what to call the person receiving mental health services. Advocates at the time reacted negatively to the label of "patient," believing it perpetuated medical-model, one-down status. "Consumer" was offered as an alternative, reflecting the choice people have when engaging in services. "Client" was the status quo term. Results showed consumer to be least endorsed as a way that people with lived experience want to be referred. A little less than half chose client. Almost a quarter had no preference. One in five chose patient.

What about leadership of the movement? Might they have stature in making these decisions? This begs the question who exactly is the movement and who are their leaders? Unlike the National Alliance on Mental Illness (NAMI), an advocacy group made up mostly of parents of adult children with serious mental illness, no single group has clearly come to represent the perspective of people with lived experience themselves. Still, shouldn't advocates be sensitive to words? If a person wants the label to be "mental health challenge," then yes, others should try to respect their choice. But this is not always such an easy choice. The term schizophrenic is anathema to most advocates. Yet, Schizophrenics Anonymous is a six-step program for people with schizophrenia that had at one time grown to more than 150 chapters in the United States as well as Australia, Brazil, Canada, Mexico, and India. Might we be unaccepting to them and their group if we deny their choice of the term schizophrenic? I admit, it is a little shrill for me. But then, there are gays who choose to call themselves faggots. Granted, in part this is an in-your-face way of hitting homophobia in the face. But simple solutions about what can and cannot be said are by no means easy.

STIGMA IS A STIGMATIZING WORD

An especially ironic word concern is that the word *stigma* worsens preju-dice and discrimination. Referring to our activity as "stigma change" might undermine our goals. Several reasons are commonly provided. Some believe stigma blames people for the prejudice and discrimination heaped on them by their community. Their argument is based on the Greek translation of stigma (στίγμα) as "mark," interpreting the idea as mark being characteris-tic of the person and blaming them for the characteristic. Erving Goffman (1963) is often credited for reintroducing "stigma" into the modern era, equating it with mark or cue. But stigma as outlined by Goffman exceeds narrow understanding of characteristic. Instead, stigma is a social process launched by a cue. It includes prejudice and discrimination evoked by cues: skin color, body features, or prostheses. Labels and diagnoses are the marks leading to mental illness stigma. Nowhere in this equation does Goffman suggest people are responsible for their marks. In fact, he quite clearly admits stigma is a blemish of the society in which it festers. The stigmatizer is the focus of stigma change. Nowhere does credible research imply that people with mental illness are to blame for their marks.

A second critique is the belief that the term "stigma" is solely used for mental illness. After all, the prejudice of color, gender, age, and sexual ori-entation are known as racism, sexism, ageism, and homophobia; no "stigma" here. This is selective perception, however. Doctor Martin Luther King, Jr. in his 1968 speech at Grosse Point High School outside Detroit said:

you failed to realize that America made the black man's color a stigma. Something that he couldn't change. Not only was the color a stigma, but even linguistic then stigmatic conspired against the black man so that his color was thought of as something very evil.

(King Jr., 1968)

One might respond that although eloquent, Dr. King's words are almost fifty years old. The message remains poignant. In 2005, the Institute for Research on Poverty at the University of Wisconsin–Madison published a report titled *Racial Stigma and Its Consequences* (Loury, 2005).

Others criticize "stigma" saying it is applied to psychiatric disorders but not other physical illnesses. This is also incorrect. I am editor of *Stigma and Health* published by the American Psychological Association. In the past two years, I have reviewed more than 150 manuscripts on stigma. Sure, mental illness is there, but it rests among concerns about the stigma of cancer, HIV-AIDS, hearing loss, and Moebius syndrome. In fact, the most manuscripts submitted to the journal have been on weight and obesity, not mental illness.

Opponents to "stigma" want to replace the term with "prejudice" and "discrimination," arguing they are more explanatory of harmful social processes. Of course they are; Goffman said that in his 1963 book. So what is the harm of eliminating the term? Here, I think those against the term show ignorance of social linguistics. The choir may be sensitive to the nuance. But the average person, he or she who might discriminate against people with a mental illness label, does not care about abolishing the term. I had one research participant say to me, "Stigma is what harms people with mental illness. I don't know about this other stuff." Of course, other words prominent in everyday language have been set aside; what about stigma? Research has this question in a study of 340 members drawn from the "normal" majority who were exposed to a vignette about Harry, an employed, middle-aged man with schizophrenia (Sheehan et al., 2016). The vignette ends with the statement, "He [Harry] sometimes worries that he will experience [stigma/prejudice/reactions] from his co-workers," with research participants randomly assigned to one of these three terms. If concerns about stigma as a stigmatizing term were correct, we would expect stigma to be viewed as a more disrespectful term than prejudice. No such difference was found. Even more, "reactions," another term preferred to stigma, was actually viewed as more disrespectful.

In 2014, I joined the Committee on Science of Changing Behavioral Health Social Norms, hosted by the National Academy of Sciences and funded by SAMHSA. Our efforts led to the National Academies of Sciences (NAS; 2016) release, *Ending Discrimination Against People with Mental and Substance Use Disorders: The Evidence for Stigma Change*, where we proposed five recommendations to guide the national agenda for stigma reduction. At the first meeting, a SAMHSA official told the committee that they—the government—had decided as policy that "stigma" was a forbidden word, that they had struck it from all present and future documents, and that they wanted us to heed this concern in our work. As an aside, I had worked with a colleague with lived experience who submitted a presentation titled *Changing Stigma Through Disclosure* to the SAMHSA-funded Alternatives Conference. She was excited when it was accepted but dismayed when she attended the conference only to find out that "stigma" had been edited out of the program. I was outraged. This was another example of an all-knowing bureaucrat telling the little guy with lived experience that she was ignorant.

Regardless of my scholarly talents, I responded to the SAMHSA official with my Irish sense of independence. "I am sorry but I have not worked in this area for more than 15 years to allow some bureaucrats to dictate to me how I will speak about this topic." She responded that prejudice and discrimination were better terms. I don't disagree that stigma is prejudice and discrimination. But you don't get rid of stigma by striking it from the vernacular. The average person understands what stigma is—it is what happens to people with undesirable health conditions. Prejudice and discrimination—that is what happens to black people.

Walking tiptoe around words leads to the kind of bureaucratic speak of government officials. Just look at the NAS committee's name: Changing Behavioral Health *Social Norms*. Alan Leshner, past CEO of the American Association for the Advancement of Science, called out this government speak at an NAS-sponsored people

(*continued*)

meeting on stigma in 2015. To paraphrase, Leshner said, "Social norms. What are those? If you mean stigma, just say stigma."

Surgeon General Vivek Murthy in the preface of his 2016 report *Facing Addiction in America* said,

> For far too long, too many in our country have viewed addiction as a moral failing. This unfortunate *stigma* has created an added burden of shame that has made people with substance use disorders less likely to come forward and seek help.

SAMHSA's principal administrator, Kana Enomoto, wrote the foreword to the Surgeon's Report. I guess she didn't get the anti-stigma message from Dr. Murthy.

Is this how we want to spend our time, fighting among ourselves on something as trivial as words? We want to organize into an effective force to help those unaware of stigma's harmful effects promote affirming attitudes. Chastising someone on inappropriate words does not help.

The final argument about stigma being a stigmatizing word is a distaste of programs focusing on stigma. They are another example of focus on the bad and broken associated with mental illness, a perspective that often emerges from psychiatry. The goal should be to promote recovery and self-determination. Of course it is. Hence, we stress that programs need to yield affirming attitudes and behaviors. As said earlier, social justice related to race is advanced only when the "N" word is replaced by rightful opportunities at all levels of society. Similar goals apply to mental illness; communities that foster recovery and self-determination for people with serious mental illness are the gold standard. Black activists realize, however, that the stigma of race continues to block opportunity. Sometimes, progressives might think we have surpassed the time of racism so that all that remains is implementing social justice. The Black Lives Matter's agenda of the past few years decries this naiveté. In like manner, as we pursue recovery and self-determination, we need to be aware that the stigma of mental illness continues and that programs meant to tear it down are necessary parallels to those that enhance affirming goals.

WHO OWNS THE WORDS?

Sometimes, advocates compare stigma and stigma change of people with mental illness to that experienced by the LGBT community. One way advocates and researchers have called for erasing the stigma of mental illness is for people to come out; like those in the gay community, people with serious mental illness strategically decide to share their stories of recovery, demanding empowerment and solidarity in the process. The value of coming out for mental illness is discussed more fully in chapter 7.

Some people in the LGBT community have reacted in anger. Partly, they are concerned that this message is another attempt to pathologize being LGBT as the psychiatric profession has done for more than one hundred years. (Although the American Psychiatric Association decided to remove homosexuality from the DSM-III in 1973, some version of deviance remained for many years after, such as "ego dystonic homosexuality." Most would now agree that pathologized versions of LGBT are absent from the 2013 edition of DSM-5). Anything that suggests LGBT is a symptom of mental illness is anathema to their goals, a view I agree with. As a result, some of the LGBT community bristle at the idea of people with mental illness coming out.

Advocacy groups need to be careful in asserting proprietorship over words and concepts. Coming out has had great value as an idea for advancing a gay agenda. Advocates, however, do not serve broader goals of social justice when they assert coming out is theirs alone to use. Would this assertion mean that the gay agenda owns the idea of closet? What about shame, or stigma, or prejudice? The power of gay rights gained ascendancy when the population realized this is another example of the progressive ideal—no element of social life should ever limit a group of people because of stigma. Even more, LGBT advocates need to make sure they are not perpetuating stigma in their own right, namely, the idea that a lesbian is not as bad as a woman with schizophrenia. Social justice is advanced by partnership, not bickering.

BEATING STIGMA IS MORE THAN
CHANGING WORDS

There are unintended consequences when advocates prioritize word change in order to beat stigma. First, diagnostic relabeling focuses stigma change within the professions and not among people with lived experience. This might be a good place to start given mental health practitioners are among the most stigmatizing of trades, careers, and vocations (Schulze, 2007). Many psychiatrists, for example, often endorse stereotypes about mental illness, including dangerousness and incompetence, or do not believe recovery is a legitimate model of serious disorders like schizophrenia (Torrey, 2011). Despite its promise, diagnostic relabeling in order to change stigma entangles the issue in the medical perspective and its misguided notions of prognosis and recovery.

The power of changing the diagnostic name of schizophrenia is linked by some psychiatrists to "lasting recovery if treated with therapy and psychosocial care" (Sartorius et al., 2014). This suggests recovery is achieved and stigma is lessened when the person deals with disease according to these prescriptions. It might follow, therefore, that people who are not adhering to professional recommendations are worsening stigma. In addition, a focus on diagnostic relabeling shows misunderstanding of the endurance of prejudice and discrimination. Some might say stigma is erased when people stop acting mentally ill (Torrey, 2011). Whether people with serious mental illness are diagnosed with schizophrenia, or a more benign and informed label like integration disorder, they are still labeled. The person is still marked as different. The harm of stigma arises from both the mark and the difference.

Finally, a focus on diagnostic relabeling misrepresents the direction between language and stigma. The term schizophrenia is not what leads to stigma; stigma is what causes shame as a result of the schizophrenia label. Relabeling disrespectful terms for serious mental illness might yield short-term effects so that the "normal" majority view the condition with less stigma. But eventually, pairing new terms with a condition that continues to be stigmatized by a culture will stain that term too.

STIGMA CHANGE IS EASY

Focusing on words makes anti-stigma efforts seem easy; all we need do in order to stop the discrimination is change the words. Believing stigma change is easy has its consequences. Funding bodies like the National Institute of Mental Health vary priorities so that support for research in stigma has waxed and waned over the past decade. Believing stigma has changed with words, professional groups opine it is time to leave the agendas of anti-stigma programs behind (Rosenberg, 2013).

In chapter 2, *slacktivism* was presented as one way in which word change gains strength as an anti-stigma agenda. Slacktivism is a set of feel-good measures meant to support a social cause that has no meaningful effect. It is often seen in social media where people like, share, or tweet a cause to promote its social justice intent. Little effort is required and little impact is realized. Addressing stigma through word work yields the same feel-good fecklessness. Changing words distracts the "normal" majority from the hard work needed to change public and self-stigma.

BEWARE WORD POLICE

Word work also leads to word police, people who are ready to pull a discussion to the side of the road in order to set straight the person with misguided terms. Advocacy efforts get derailed in this atmosphere. One colleague of mine said it well:

> I don't care what you call it. We just need to make sure people stop robbing me of my life goals because of my mental health history.

This sense of derailment is even worse for people not immersed in the stigma world. The choir of advocates might be patient with the search for appropriate language. But the people we want to change, those in the "normal" majority who are not aware of stigma's harm, are not going to understand, or care about, the subtlety of this discussion.

Advocates need to understand the effects of don't: "don't think this, don't say that!" This kind of protest leads to unintended consequences discussed more in chapter 5. Briefly, psychological reactance is a fundamental process; people rebel against dictums telling them what to do. Research reviewed in chapter 5 shows telling the "normal" majority "not to stigmatize those with mental illness" leads to a rebound effect that makes things worse. The same thing happens to word police. The "normal" majority are likely to dismiss the zealot who lectures them on appropriate language. This parallels an important principle in anti-stigma research. "Don't stigmatize the stigmatizer." Don't say, "Shame on you for thinking bad things about people with mental illness!" It is unlikely that those who endorse prejudice and discriminate do so willingly or consciously. Disparaging "stigmatizers" only makes them defensive. Word police who spank people for their uninformed use of words fan these flams. Instead, we want to make the "normal" majority partners with advocates in our joint agenda to promote social justice.

Still, might not word police have some legitimacy in the face of egregious words? I would correct someone using the "N" word or "R" word without hesitation, because society agrees that these words have no place in our world. Although research has not been done per se on the degree to which the "normal" majority agrees these words have no place in our world, it is reasonable to believe population studies would bear out these assumptions. What about mental health? Is there not some agreement among research about ways of referring to people with mental illness? This question has been the focus of numerous studies; I was part of a group that searched for consensus on ways to refer to people with mental illness more than twenty years ago (Mueser, Glynn, Corrigan, & Baber, 1996). The term "patient" was common in the medical community at the time but viewed negatively with advocates instead urging use of terms like client or consumer. Results failed to show any one term was significantly more preferred than the others. While 45 percent of participants liked the term client, consumer was endorsed by just 8 percent with patient in between at 27 percent. Research since then has echoed these findings, even when comparison terms change; e.g., what is the value of person first language? There is no consensus. We concluded our 1996 paper with a recommendation that remains today. Stigma and harm is an individual experience. Hence, we should look to individuals with mental illness as to how they wish to be known. Individual perspectives differ. Therefore, we should be respectful of this difference and accept the individual's way of understanding his or her experience. Word police undermine this goal.

IS THIS OUR BEST SHOT?

Americans are hit from many sides with new perspectives on social justice. I am amazed at a few that I have been trying to understand over the past few years. Should transgender people be allowed to use bathrooms of their choice? Gender is not a categorical phenomenon but rather fluid. Do my courses need trigger warnings? The average member of the general public is not waiting for another effort to change their beliefs and actions about a group. They have limited cognitive resources. That's why advocates need to consider their approaches judiciously; what is the best way to make people aware of an anti-stigma agenda that helps them move to more affirming attitudes and actions as a result?

We need to keep our mind on the target. People who are allies and reading this book are those who are going to care about whether to call it stigma or discrimination or whatever. They are not our target. It is the average people, the masses, whose opinions we seek to change—people like my Aunt Lillian who spent most of her adult life working at the A&P supermarket chain in Chicago. She does not get this finely nuanced discussion nor would she care. Let us not waste her time on a politically correct distraction. The next three chapters review well-researched approaches to stigma change—protest, education, and contact—in light of their strengths and unintended consequences.

5

PROTEST: JUST SAY NO TO STIGMA

ROTEST COMES TO mind when striving to correct social injustice, people organizing into articulate movements of dissent. We proudly recall Martin Luther King Jr., leading the march across the Pettus Bridge into Selma, Alabama, to replace Jim Crow laws with rights guaranteed by the U.S. Constitution. The Vietnam War bumped against college students who wanted none of it: "Hey, hey, LBJ. We don't want no war today!" One might think, therefore, that protest would be the place to begin shutting down the stigma of mental illness so people with these labels have rights for them to achieve personal goals. Protest addresses the rights agenda. It seeks to remove barriers so people with mental illness can pursue rightful opportunities related to work, education, independent living, and other social arenas.

Protest, however, seems to have unintended consequences (the stigma effect) that may undercut its value as an anti-stigma approach, especially when seeking to change stereotypical attitudes in which discrimination rests. These consequences are reviewed here. Still, protest may have some value in targeting media representations of people with mental illness. Television and movie producers may, at times, respond to concerted efforts of advocates who have organized as a market force against disrespectful images. Possible strengths of this form of protest are considered.

PROTEST AND ATTITUDE REBOUND

Our research group has carefully contrasted protest's effects on stigma change compared to education. In this work, program participants are exposed to disrespectful images, often taken from the news media.

FREED MENTAL PATIENT KILLS MOM

From the *New York Post*.

GET THE VIOLENT CRAZIES OFF THE STREETS

From the *New York Daily News*.

Participants are then told the obvious—that these are shameful and hence unacceptable views that need to end. "Stop thinking that way!" Protest is an appeal to some kind of moral authority to suppress wrong thoughts. Social science, however, has shown that instruction to suppress attitudes often leads to a rebound effect. Consider this self-test often used in Intro to Psychology classes: For the next two minutes, do *not* think about white bears.

I bet most readers have some version of the Klondike bear bouncing around their head. Instructing someone *not* to think something actually increases that thought; this is an assertion that has been tested in stigma research. Instructing someone *not* to think bad things about a group actually makes attitudes about that group worse. Social psychologists have tested this in laboratory research where participants were told to suppress stereotypes about photographed skinheads (Macrae, Bodenhausen, Milne, & Jetten, 1994) or male hairdressers (Macrae, Bidenhausen, & Milne, 1998). Subsequently, research participants freely recalled more stereotypes about targets or distanced themselves from them in a discriminatory way. We did a similar study where research participants were given a photograph of a person labeled as mentally ill and told not to think bad things about that person. Results were mixed, but it seemed like attitudes got worse (Penn & Corrigan, 2002). These findings might be explained by psychological reactance, that is, people respond negatively to situations where their beliefs are perceived as being limited. It is a fundamentally American way of responding: "Don't tell me what to think." Psychological reactance is worse when recommendations seem to come from an authority. Hence, there is a general suspicion of recommendations made by government-led authorities. If the anti-stigma goal is to change attitudes of a community group, chastising them to not think that way will only make it worse.

PROTESTING A MEDIA BEHAVIOR

Sometimes protest occurs in a manner reminiscent of the 1960s—segments of the community, joined by allies, organize against disrespectful images. Consider, for example, 1960s and 1970s campaigns to stop using Aunt Jemima and Little Black Sambo as marketing tools. Aunt Jemima emerged from black-faced minstrel shows that idealized antebellum plantation life. One entrepreneur used Aunt Jemima to host a chain of pancake houses across the United States beginning in the 1950s. At the same time, a restaurant called Sambo's emerged. The Sambo story was about a South Indian boy who had lively adventures with four tigers of the jungle. Social critics including Langston Hughes criticized the story as popularizing the notion of pickaninnies, overly solicitous black children. Blacks, along with allies from other ethnic groups, joined in moratoria against the restaurants until they either ceased using the image or replaced it with a more respectful narrative.

Advocates have tried similar protests against stigmatizing images of people with mental illness. In 2000, ABC launched a TV show called *Wonderland* set in a prison ward of a psychiatric hospital in Manhattan. In its first episode, a person with mental illness shot at five police officers and stabbed a pregnant psychiatrist in the abdomen with a hypodermic needle. Needless to say, advocates were concerned and contacted producers to recommend toning down violence in the show. Prominent among these was StigmaBusters, an online community hosted by the National Alliance on Mental Illness, which sponsors e-mail- and letter-writing campaigns against media representations that disrespect mental illness. Advocates were early in their efforts, failing to realize that any contact with producers, even negative comments, says someone is watching their show. An audience is the

I am a 1960s voyeur. I was old enough to understand the power of civil rights and antiwar protests but too young to participate. I was twelve in 1968 when college students occupied Grant Park in Chicago to disrupt the Democratic National Convention. But I did not participate, as I was too young to really grasp the significance of the events. My reactions were also influenced by my Republican parents who more likely focused on those "outside violent agitators" rather than the young optimists seeking to reset the wrongs of disparity and war. But Chicago was still an amazing place for me to be at the time. Martin Luther King Jr., expanded his civil rights agenda by taking on housing discrimination in the city. I recall when he went down in the streets after being crowned on the head by a stone from an angry member of the mob. I remember two years later when four students were killed while participating in an antiwar rally at Kent State University, shot by Ohio's National Guard. Protest became wrapped up with righteousness of the innocent.

I am genetically Catholic. I went to St. Nicolas Grade School, Notre Dame High School, and Creighton University (a Jesuit school) where I learned the power of Jesus Christ in stemming the immoral with honesty and solidarity. I failed to ever find Jesus in the twentieth century. But Dr. King, and then Mahatma Gandhi, and the students in Grant Park and Kent State came very close. They were willing to advance their values even by ultimate sacrifice. And this marked me, such that I led a protest at Creighton University . . . in 1978. I was ten years too late and Creighton in Omaha, Nebraska, was never the boiling pot of dissent witnessed at Berkeley. I think the issue was less of social concern—our ROTC was hosting a public education day—and more an effort to exercise my protest skills.

My wife, Georgeen (with whom I co-led the Creighton protest), was a Cook County Public Defender. We taught our children that righting social wrong was among the most profound of vocations. My son, Abe, is now a paralegal in a law firm that addresses civil rights violations by urban police forces. My daughter, Liz, works

(continued)

with the American Red Cross at the Mexican border to set up immigration centers.

So protest is holy to me, and the natural first step for challenging the stigma of mental illness. That is why social psych research on attitude rebound surprised me, cutting my natural approach to erasing stigma at the knees. I probably overcompensated preaching that protest needs to be avoided as a strategic approach to stop stigma. Then Sally Zinman sat me down after one of my public lectures. Sally is a few years older than I am and, rather than being a voyeur, was an active protester on human rights. Sally is also a leader in the anti-stigma movement, having come out with her experiences with mental illness more than forty years ago, when discussing her time in the psych hospital was really outrageous. She appreciated my research, but was not ready to relinquish a large and organized voice calling for ending stigma. Like other civil rights heroes, Sally inspires me, leaving me to seek the best balance between protest and rebound.

greatest prize. So advocates broadened their focus by communicating with commercial sponsors of *Wonderland*, including CEOs of Mitsubishi, Sears, and the Scott Company. They realized that people with mental illness are a shopping constituency that cannot be alienated without a cost. As a result, sponsors convinced ABC management to pull the show with several episodes yet to be shown. There are recurring bad examples of Hollywood gone astray, seeking to sell movies or TV shows on the backs of disparaging images of people with mental illness. Might other concerted efforts at organizing the buying power of people against stigma be used? Perhaps not.

Psycho Donuts is a real-world commercial enterprise, with shops in Campbell and Santa Clara, California. Donuts have been named the Jasonut, Suicide Squeeze, and Crazy Face; they are "Crazy good!" Staff were dressed like Nurse Ratched, and they had a padded cell. Once again, advocates were concerned and organized an effort to address this message. Their goal was not to stop Psycho Donuts from trade but rather to tone down its message. Advocates started "a national online food fight" asking to turn "lemon donuts into lemonade." A different response was found this time. Stan Rezaee from examiner.com said it succinctly:

I'm an advocate of equal rights and a more tolerant world toward all people of different races, religion, gender, and sexual orientation: but that is it. Anything else is just moronic.

Labeling one's business as crazy, or psycho, or nuts is protected by the First Amendment. Since then, Psycho Donuts went franchise.

The First Amendment poses an interesting challenge to advocates seeking social justice. Freedom of speech is fundamental to correcting social ills; the voice of the minority needs to have full opportunity to express concerns about the status quo. The eloquence of Dr. King, in particular, led to flashbulb moments in the civil rights movement. However, these same protections permit media to express disrespectful images of people with lived experience. Moreover, boundaries between drama and disrespect are often fuzzy. Consider *Thrrteen Rzasons Why*, a 2017 Netflix series following the story of teen Hannah Baker after her death by suicide was left on several audiocassettes. Some authors in the teen genre hailed the show as an honest look at the challenges of adolescent life in these times. But many public health epidemiologists are concerned that this kind of show glorifies suicide, leading to contagion among high school students. There is no simple resolution.

THE AMERICANS WITH DISABILITIES ACT

Sometimes the effects of protest are institutionalized by acts of the legislature. This is essentially what culminated into the Civil Rights Act of 1965 championed by Lyndon B. Johnson. The works of Martin Luther King Jr., and colleagues in the South produced what is considered the landmark voting rights act of American history, assuring people of color had all privileges set out in the Fourteenth and Fifteenth Amendments of the Constitution. Similarly, George H.W. Bush signed the Americans with

Disabilities Act (ADA) of 1990, which sought to eliminate discrimination in five areas: employment, transportation, telecommunication, public accommodation, and the business of local and state government. Its application in the workplace had especially important ramifications for people with mental illness. The ADA prohibits discrimination in all phases of employment. It provides protection to "qualified individuals with disabilities"; that is, individuals with disabilities are qualified to perform the "essential functions" of an employment position. If an individual with a disability requires "reasonable accommodation" to perform the work, then employers covered under the law are required to make this accommodation, provided it does not cause "undue hardship," defined as an "action requiring significant difficulty or expense for the business" determined on the basis of factors such as the cost of the accommodation and the employer's financial resources.

The ADA was the product of years of coordinated activity and protest led by, among other people, Justin Dart. Dart is often viewed as the Martin Luther King Jr., of the disability rights movement. He had significant ambulatory difficulties as a result of childhood polio that required lifelong use of a wheelchair. In 1988, Dart launched the Road to Freedom Tour with his wife, Yoshiko. They set out to visit all fifty states promoting disability rights—no small feat since wheelchair accessibility was greatly limited at the time. During that time, he joined several advisory groups of the federal government including the National Council on Disability and the President's Committee on Employment of People with Disabilities, gaining the ear of Congress and the president for national legislation guaranteeing the rights of Americans with disabilities. He sat next to President Bush in the Rose Garden when the president signed the bill in 1990. Mr. Dart received the Presidential Medal of Freedom from Bill Clinton in 1998.

ADA's impact for psychiatric disability was not immediately evident in 1990. The legislation was in place for five years before anyone ever thought to apply it to psychiatric disabilities; the Equal Employment Opportunities Commission released a directive so stipulating in 1995. Examples of psychiatric impairments requiring accommodation include difficulties in concentrating, dealing with stress, and interacting with other people. The ADA also makes it illegal during the preemployment process to ask questions about the nature or severity of a disability. For example, an employer cannot ask job applicants about their psychiatric history.

The courts are often the place to formally protest injustice. The *Olmstead v. L.C.* case referred to a Georgia lawsuit filed on behalf of two women with intellectual and psychiatric disabilities who were inpatients in a state psychiatric hospital. Although hospital staff all agreed that the women were ready for discharge, they remained hospitalized because no appropriate community placements were available. In 1999 the U.S. Supreme Court considered the case, which involved interpreting a regulation in the ADA, which states:

> A public entity shall administer services, programs, and activities in the most integrated setting appropriate to the needs of qualified individuals with disabilities.
>
> (28 C.F.R.§ 35.130(d))

The Court ruled that the unnecessary segregation of individuals with disabilities in institutions may constitute discrimination based on disability. This decision has been interpreted as requiring the community placement of institutional residents when the state's own treating professionals have recommended such placement.

WHERE WAS DR. KING'S STATISTICIAN?

Dr. Marin Luther King Jr., accomplished historic change in social justice for African Americans without social science outcome research. Before him, Mahatma Gandhi taught peaceful civil disobedience as a cure to imperialism without population researchers. They did this without findings from social science. No one calls them naïve. Their dedication and impact inspire progressively minded people who charge into the social injustice of stigma. Resolving a social wrong seems more a matter of righteous morality than empirical study. This is a humbling realization for me when wearing my scientist's hat. Are the rigors of research really helpful here?

I am not yet ready to discard empirical investigation altogether. I have learned important, unexpected lessons from my research that inform this book. But research cannot be a drag on advocacy efforts. Scientists cannot tell advocates to wait patiently while we collect evidence that discerns effective from ineffective approaches. The worth of our research lies with its ability to inform and arm advocates in their efforts to replace stigma with affirming attitudes and actions—the advocate's imperative. This does not mean all research needs to test the effects of anti-stigma programs; basic investigations have their value. But it does mean research needs to have some manifest relevance to changing the public discussion leading to less stigma.

6

BEWARE THE EDUCATIONAL FIX

T HERE ARE TWO major messages I wish to leave the reader, mentioned earlier, but detailed in chapters 6 and 7. They are meant to be first principles in what I think are directions for replacing stigma with affirming attitudes. First, I argue in this chapter that education, at least for adults, is an overrated, mostly feckless approach to erasing stigma. In some ways, the educational zeal of the Western world is the biggest example of the stigma effect. Second, I present in the next chapter the effective alternative—contact with people in recovery. Education is built on a basic premise that knowledge is the opposite of the ignorance, which leads to prejudice and discrimination. This seems almost to be a truism. But seeking to promote knowledge through education to decrease stigma is rarely effective. Westerners are infatuated with education; from a historical perspective, it has advanced human opportunity exponentially over the past two hundred years. We have moved from a people working on the farm or in factories to an information-based population where more lucrative and stimulating careers are linked to learning. Our children spend longer and longer times in school to prepare them for satisfying vocations and lucrative jobs. Education exposes students to deeper and broader perspectives on other groups, undermining a sense of difference that is at the heart of stereotype and prejudice. Prejudice is replaced by acceptance and opportunity. Public health-and-safety experts use education to advance knowledge about health challenges and evidence-based ways to prevent or treat them.

Therefore, a "normal" majority that better understands mental illness is less likely to view them as different. Comprehension of evidence-based treatments might replace fear of the mentally ill with optimism that they are peers who can become full members of society.

Scientific positivism blossomed in the early nineteenth century as an optimistic epistemology in which knowledge has certainly expanded for researchers and professionals through the empirical method. Educational positivism is its conceptual peer, that the public as a whole is better able to access this knowledge base through planned pedagogic endeavors. Both are fundamentally hopeful and democratic; i.e., that anyone with sufficient training can access what is known about illness in order to promote health. Scientific positivism, however, was shown to be incomplete leading to critical evolutions, that not everything can be known through the scientific method. Educational positivism also has its limits. At its extreme, educational positivism leads to a "more is better" confidence that often leads to overwhelming education programs. Several well-intentioned educational programs seem to worsen stigma. After a brief review of education formats, unintended consequences of education programs are described.

EDUCATION AND PUBLIC STIGMA

Education is often used to address the services agenda. Namely, with better understanding of symptoms and treatment, the "normal" majority is more willing to ignore stigma and become engaged in care. What does an education program targeting the stigma of mental illness look like? They often contrast myths of mental illness (believed to be the basis of stereotypes) with facts (that emerge from research).

MYTH: People choose to be mentally ill.
FACT: Serious mental illness is largely biological in origin.

This is the personal responsibility myth, which has been clearly discredited by modern neuroscience. Studies consistently show serious psychoses such as schizophrenia are attributable to genetics or in utero insult. People do not choose to be psychotic because of lack of moral backbone.

MYTH: People with serious mental illness are dangerous and unpredictable.

FACT: They are more likely to be victims of crime than perpetrators.

I unpacked the complexities of the dangerous myth in chapter 2 where I concluded that the "normal" majority overestimates the level of dangerousness among people with mental illness by tenfold or more, an estimate that balloons soon after one of the mass shootings haunting American culture.

MYTH: Serious mental illness is rare.

FACT: Many, many people are in recovery from serious mental illness.

I call this the leprosy myth. Christians learned in the New Testament that leprosy was this scourge handed down by God to a small group of dirty, punished people. The key point here is SMALL group, that somehow, because leprosy harms only a handful of people it represents the rare and watchful eye of a vengeful god. Mental illness is the same kind of plague, harm wrought on this tiny segment of an unkempt population. After all, it seems like few of us know someone with an illness. In reality, serious mental illness is common in the adult population with as many as 20 percent meeting criteria for diagnoses in their adult years. Consider the prototype "bad" illness, schizophrenia, to put this into better perspective. Research shows about 0.8 percent of the population meets criteria for schizophrenia, a seemingly tiny number until we do the math. In the Chicago metropolitan area, that's 80,000 people, more than two-thirds of the population of our state capital, Springfield. People in Chicago are likely to regularly interact with individuals with schizophrenia at work, on the train, or in church but just not realize it.

MYTH: People with mental illness are incapable of serious vocations or meaningful jobs.

FACT: People with mental illness are represented in all levels of careers.

In some ways, this myth represents falsehoods about recovery; namely, that people with serious mental illness are unable to live with their disabilities and pursue the full range of life goals. This myth robs people of hope and self-determination.

EDUCATION'S APPEAL

Educational approaches are popular because they are easy to develop and disseminate. A group of well-intentioned advocates can quickly put together an education program by combing the research literature about key facts and misunderstandings about mental illness and treatment. The educational program is then paired with action statements—take-home messages meant to move affirming attitudes and actions, for example, encouraging people to seek help when depressed or anxious. Educational programs are often translated into pencil-and-paper manuals that advocacy groups disseminate across a country along with simple train-the-trainer manuals. In this way, large portions of a population can be exposed to the program and its goals.

Educational programs are further advanced when embedded in social marketing campaigns. Social marketing represents the strategic use of economic and social forces in order to change behaviors that lead to social problems (Kotler, Roberto, & Lee, 2002). Social marketing learns from commercialism. Both have a customer focus. The target of change is a market sector that is defined in terms of social exchange between the group in control of marketing and the group whose behavior is the focus of change. These sectors are segmented; the effectiveness of marketing depends on defining relevant sectors and then crafting a marketing format that reflects the sectors' needs and interests. Customers of both efforts must perceive the benefits of partaking in the product or behavior as exceeding the costs of engaging in a different behavior. Still, there are notable differences between social and commercial marketing. They differ in terms of goals. Commercial marketing promotes sellable products or services crafted for targeted groups. The product in social marketing is behavior change. In public health campaigns, for example, this includes abandoning old behaviors (stop-smoking efforts), rejecting harmful behavior (to moderate future substance use), and accepting new behaviors (health and wellness). Indicators of success differ as a result. The goals of commercial marketing are financial and seek to maximize profit. Social marketing addresses social problems through behavior change of the market group. Approaches also vary in terms of competition. Competition in commercial marketing is the other companies or organizations that sell similar products. Competition in social marketing is the status quo behaviors that keep a group from diminishing the social problem.

PUBLIC SERVICE ANNOUNCEMENTS

Public service campaigns are prominent examples of social marketing and education. The Substance Abuse and Mental Health Administration (SAMHSA) has been a major force in anti-stigma adopting public service campaigns. Public service announcements (PSAs) are a media-based core to public service campaigns. In 2004, SAMHSA launched the Campaign for Mental Health Recovery, a multiyear public service effort to promote social inclusion and support. SAMHSA's campaign—*What a Difference a Friend Makes*—was designed to encourage young adults to step up and support friends living with mental health problems. The campaign launched nationally in December 2006 and included television, radio, outdoor, print, and web elements, as well as a printed brochure and website. TV and radio components were distributed to over 28,000 media outlets nationwide.

An especially poignant PSA—*Be There!*—had two young men sitting next to each other in a darkened room playing a computer game. They appear uncomfortable, stealing sidelong looks at each other. **Voice-over:** "It can be a little awkward when your friend tells you he's been diagnosed with a mental illness. But what's even more awkward is if you're not there for him, he's less likely to recover." **GUY 2 then says:** "I'm here to help, man. Whatever it takes." The PSA fades to the website. This is actually SAMHSA's second anti-stigma campaign with PSAs; the first was called the *Elimination of Barriers Initiative* (EBI), a three-year pilot begun with eight states in 2003. The scene in one of its PSAs—*Part of Our Lives*—showed "regular people" (a storeowner, a mother of two, and an honor student) with voice-over that states all the people shown have "recovered from a mental illness." It ended with the phone number of the National Mental Health Consumers' Self-Help Clearinghouse and its Internet address.

Another PSA, released on October 21, 2009, featured film star Glenn Close. Set in a large train station, pairs of actors wear light-colored T-shirts, half of them labeled in blue print with a mental illness. They are partnered with a person labeled as a loved one. One man's shirt says "schizophrenia," and next to him in a similar shirt is "mom." Another person's shirt says "bipolar" and is paired with "better half." Glenn Close's shirt reads "sister," standing next to her is real-life sister Jessie with "bipolar" on her shirt. There are definite benefits to this kind of PSA. Close's star power, for example, had significant effects as evidenced by the news and online activity created by the PSA. While respecting Ms. Close's intention, this is an excellent example of an unintended PSA. What does the viewer see? People reduced to labels. There are the labels of the mentally ill—schizophrenia and bipolar disorder—and of normal people. The "normal" majority is able to assume important life roles: mom, partner, sister. People with lived experience are not.

There are few published studies evaluating American PSA efforts for mental illness despite ample research supported by the federal government on PSA effects on smoking and HIV/AIDS (DeJong, Wolf, & Austin, 2001; Goldman & Glantz, 1998). These other studies led to guidelines for measuring PSA effects understood as assessing penetration or impact. Consider how penetration is assessed on product marketing; Coca-Cola designs a dancing pop can as a way to gain market attention for its product. Penetration is a function of recall and recognition memory; does the "normal" majority remember ever seeing the dancing can on TV, the Internet, or in print ads? Do people remember seeing or hearing a specific anti-stigma PSA? Consider this self-test as one way to assess PSA effects. Ask how many people in a group of acquaintances recall seeing SAMHSA or Glenn Close PSAs. This task is recollection; namely, with minor cues can the person repeat back some aspect of a PSA? Alternatively, measures assess whether people are able to recognize a TV ad or radio jingle when presented to them. Third, regardless of recall or recognition, what gist of the PSA can be repeated? What part of the PSA message can the person retell? PSA penetration should lead to some recall, recognition, and gist.

PSAs need to be observable in the public to penetrate the population. One evaluation showed the EBI *Part of Our Lives* was sent to 627 television organizations in eight pilot states, 62 percent of broadcast outlets and 225 cable systems (Bell, Colangelo, & Pillen, 2005). For radio stations, 3671 received radio kits, which was 100 percent of English-speaking stations. Distributing PSAs is not synonymous with exposure; clearly, receipt of *Part of Our Lives* did not mean stations aired it. Actual airtime might be assessed by media organization pledges, the frequency of stations that promised to use the PSA. Twenty percent of stations that received EBI campaign materials pledged to air the PSA at least once, 6 percent of radio stations.

PSAs must penetrate a population to impact it. In product marketing, how did recalling the dancing Coke translate into increased sales? Instead of sales, PSA impact is judged by action. Did the viewer, for example, surf to a "learn more about it" website after seeing the PSA? Research on *Part of Our Lives* provided monthly website visits from November 2004 to July 2005 (Bell, Colangelo, & Pillen, 2005). Visits to the site tripled from 2,743 to 7,627 during this time and increased from 1,158 to 2,614 unique visitors. However, 88 percent of visitors exited the website in less than one minute. Fewer than 30 percent of visitors returned to the site in the subsequent months. Is an increase from 2,743 to 7,627 a significant and meaningful improvement? The different scores yield an odds ratio of 2.81, highly significant and supporting assertions about greater website hits after PSA distribution. Size of effect, however, is quite small. U.S. Census data as of July 2008 reported 124.6 million residents in the eight pilot states. That means .000061 percent of people in these states visited the website. Of course, frequency of website visits is likely to be higher when overall population in those states is reduced by, for example, percent of population that actually watched television every day (conservatively estimated at 66.0 percent according to AC Nielsen 2009 data). That increases Web visits to .000093 percent, which is still miniscule in effect.

PROBLEMS WITH PSAs

Why might PSA impact be so limited? Consider distribution in American media outlets. The Federal Communications Commission mandates that broadcast stations using the public airwaves must serve the "public interest, convenience, and necessity." One way television networks do this is as vehicles for PSAs that provide potential avenues for addressing mental health and anti-stigma agenda. Unfortunately, these opportunities are limited by when or how often PSAs are aired. Campaigns focused on mental health must compete with PSAs that consider other prominent issues, e.g., child welfare, breast cancer, and military veterans, each with important messages. PSAs are often broadcasted at off hours (2 to 4 A.M.) when fewer people are watching TV. Even if PSAs receive airtime, they are often pulled quickly from the air because PSA producers have contractual relationships with actors that stipulate the length of time in which the video may be broadcast, often one year. Distributors have to pay residuals to actors in cases when the PSA is used beyond the year. Given that PSAs are produced and distributed using charitable donations and/or public funds, additional monies to keep them on the air are often unavailable.

Still, PSAs seemed to have had major influence on impacting smoking and HIV/AIDS. What's the difference? The action messages of anti-stigma PSAs are much more difficult to pose concisely. PSA's action for smoking: stop smoking. HIV/AIDS: safe sex. I don't mean to say realizing smoking and HIV goals are easy, but communicating the focus can be done simply and efficiently. What's the goal for anti-stigma PSAs: don't? Don't be a bigot? First, this will have little effect because biased members of the "normal" majority never recognize themselves in the group of bigots. Second, even if the PSA gets their attention, what does it mean to stop being a bigot? Stop discriminating against someone. "But I don't discriminate now." Some anti-stigma programs promote affirming actions instead. SAMHSA's *Be There!* Campaign does this nicely by promoting support among friends. When peers are troubled, be there for them.

As in protest, PSA impact has been shown to boomerang. One study examined the impact of a print add (Lienemann, Siegel, & Crano, 2013). "You are not to blame for the cause of your depression. Depression is treatable if you are willing to seek help." The bottom half of the advertisement then listed indicators of depression: persistent sad mood, feelings of hopelessness, and decreased energy. Benefits might include viewers being more open to help-seeking. Results, however, were the reverse. People who saw this ad were more likely to endorse the self-stigma of depression.

Direct-to-consumer advertising (DTCA) uses marketing strategies to undermine stigma and promote product sales. DTCA for prescription medications exploded after the U.S. Food and Drug Administration (FDA) lifted restrictions in 1985. American media has been pelted by DTCA for antidepressants; DTCA revenue for Cymbalta, an antidepressant medication manufactured by Eli Lilly, was ranked fifth among all medications in 2008 (Singer, 2009). One study examining the impact of a Cymbalta advertisement demonstrated the complexity of DTCA effects (Corrigan, Kosyluk, Fokuo, & Park, 2014). The advertisement showcased seven people (men and women from diverse ethnic backgrounds) struggling with depression, mentioned the benefits of Cymbalta as an antidepressant, summarized possible physical and psychiatric side effects, and ended with people seemingly better. Unintended effects were found on public stigma. Namely, people were less likely to endorse recovery or self-determination after seeing the Cymbalta advertisement. However, if people had lived experience, if they reported previous episodes of depression, the Cymbalta ad seemed to cause less blame and more support of empowerment.

Growing concern about penetration and boomerang effects has led to skepticism about PSAs, which has begun to sway big picture perspectives about anti-stigma programs. The Canadian Mental Health Commission, for example, launched its *Opening Minds* anti-stigma initiative in 2009 with a large social marketing campaign. Results of a population survey, however, showed the campaign had no measurable effect on the Canadian public (Stuart et al., 2014). As a result, the Commission jettisoned large-scale social marketing for more local and targeted strategies.

OTHER EDUCATION EFFORTS THAT FAILED

Several programs that have used government support to pursue public health goals were unable to reach them, instead resulting in unintended consequences. Drug Abuse Resistance Education (DARE) was a widely disseminated and implemented program meant to dissuade youth from engaging in substance use. Typically led by police officers, DARE educates youth about the risks of substance use disorders and ways to resist peer pressure to avoid use. At one point, DARE was in 75 percent of U.S. school districts and forty-three countries around the world. This is one of the rare times federal and local governments collected data to examine the effects of a program they supported with research done by multiple universities and research institutes. Results led the U.S. General Accounting Office, U.S. Surgeon General, and National Academy of Sciences to conclude that DARE had no measurable effect on participant attitudes and behaviors. Even more, one study from the University of Indiana in 1992 showed unintended consequences; children who completed DARE were *more* likely to use hallucinogenic drugs at follow-up (Evans & Bosworth, 1998).

Another campaign sought to change misunderstandings about vaccinations using the myth-versus-fact education approach. A significant part of the American population believes that vaccinations in infancy lead to autism. No less than Robert F. Kennedy Jr., touts this view and was appointed by President Donald Trump to a task force meant to further examine this assertion despite unyielding evidence from the Centers for Disease Control and Prevention (CDC) and FDA to the contrary. Vaccinations protect our children from diphtheria, tetanus, pertussis, polio, measles, mumps, and rubella. Unfortunately, decisions by parents believing this myth heighten significant public health risk. The CDC, for example, has shown a steady increase of measles in its epidemiologic data over the past decade, exposing unvaccinated children to significant and unnecessary health risks (Centers for Disease Control, 2017). This is especially unfair to children who are unable to be vaccinated because of genetic and other biologic intolerance to such treatment, thereby exposing them to serious risks from the public.

Public health educators have crafted education programs to address misinformation about the vaccination-autism connection. They show parents with these beliefs clearly written FDA and CDC fact sheets that summarize state-of-the-art research contradicting the "vaccination is autism" myth. Educators combine this with compelling videotape vignettes of the anguish caused by an unnecessarily sick child who ends up deathly ill after contracting a childhood illness that could have been prevented by vaccination. Pre-post research is sobering on these programs. Parents endorsing the vaccination-autism connection show no change in these attitudes over time. Even more amazing, these parents are less likely to actually vaccinate their child after training (Nyhan, Reifler, Richey, & Freed, 2014). This is another manifestation of the boomerang effect of psychological reactance discussed in chapter 4. Misinformation about health is recalcitrant in light of thoughts about "not telling me what to think." Instead, believers of the myth dig in their heels, being even more certain about the link.

MENTAL ILLNESS IS A BRAIN DISORDER

In 1990, the National Institute of Mental Health launched the decade of the brain where the Institute was trying to bring modern psychiatry into the age of neuroscience, seeking to ground understanding of diagnosis and treatment in bench science. Advocates thought this might also be the medium by which the responsibility myth is erased. People do not choose to be schizophrenic but rather are victim of a biological disease. Mental illness became branded as a "brain disorder." Several studies tested this assertion soon after the campaign launch, with the results showing especially harmful results (Read, Haslam, Sayce, & Davies, 2006). While it is true that the "normal" majority blames people with serious mental illness less after learning the genetic roots to schizophrenia, they are also likely to believe the person will not recover.

> You may look good now, but psychosis is hard-wired into your neurons. You can snap at any time.

It is lack of belief in recovery that leads employers to not hire people with mental illness, landlords to not rent to them, or primary care doctors to offer substandard care.

These findings echo concerns about a parallel educational approach: framing mental illness like any illness.

> Schizophrenia is just like diabetes. The public does not blame people for diabetes, so it should not blame people with schizophrenia.

This yields an easy slogan to ground education programs. Research, however, is less sanguine about its effects, instead showing noticeable unintended consequences (Read, Haslam, Sayce, & Davies, 2006). Not only has "mental illness just like any illness" failed to yield benefits but findings show the slogan is associated with greater perceptions of dangerousness and unpredictability. This, in turn, leads to more fear of people labeled with mental illness and desire for greater social distance: "I don't want to work alongside those people."

Over the past decades, two ongoing programs of population research provide a broader and more definitive picture of the effects of education. The first looked at the degree to which the "normal" majority agrees that mental illness is a brain disorder, that symptoms are not chosen by the person with the illness. The second examined whether this change in knowledge corresponded with improvement in stigma. A meta-analysis of sixteen population studies from around the globe examined change in knowledge and in stigma from 1990 to 2006 (Schomerus, Schwann, & Holzinger, 2012). As expected, knowledge about schizophrenia and about depression significantly increased during this time. Knowledge grew. Between 40 and 60 percent of study participants during this time learned that schizophrenia was genetically inherited; between 50 and 70 percent of participants agreed that schizophrenia was a brain disease. Despite this significant increase, impact on stigma worsened. The index of stigma here was the degree to which survey participants would accept a person with schizophrenia as a neighbor. Responses got worse with acceptance decreasing from about 50 percent in 1990 to 30 percent in 2006. Similar glum findings were found in labor with acceptance decreasing from 50 percent in 1990 to a little above 30 percent in 2006.

MENTAL HEALTH LITERACY VERSUS STIGMA CHANGE

Although education may have limited or unintended effects on stigma in adults, increasing knowledge still has value; it leads to mental health literacy. The experience of mental illness is foreign and complex to most in the "normal" majority, both those challenged by symptoms and disabilities as well as loved ones trying to make sense of these frightening experiences while providing support to the person. Evidence-based interventions are equally complex where patients need to sort costs and benefits of medical versus psychosocial interventions offered by professionals, allied health, the ministry, or peers. The impact of knowledge is especially forceful when people are early in their mental health experience. It answers the "what's happening to me" question. Labeling strange experiences can be a source of great relief.

Education programs seek to promote mental health literacy. As mentioned in chapter 3, Anthony Jorm from Australia is among the world scholars and developers of programs that address mental health literacy; he grouped educational approaches into four categories (Jorm, 2012). (1) *Whole-of-community campaigns* seeking to orient targeted populations to the treatable challenges of mental illness. *beyondblue* from his homeland is a public service campaign of this type with more than a twenty-year record of influencing Aussie actions about depression. (2) *Interventions based in educational settings.* Schools are a natural place to promote mental health literacy with curricula developed for middle school, high school, and college students. (3) *Web-based interventions.* The Internet provides a seemingly unlimited venue for promoting knowledge about what mental illness is and how to treat it. (4) As mentioned in chapter 3, *Mental Health First Aid* (MHFA) is a widely disseminated intervention meant to promote mental health in the spirit of the Red Cross's training in CPR. Typically a two-day course, MHFA begins with a review of the phenomenology and epidemiology of serious mental illnesses in the *Diagnostic and Statistical Manual of Mental Disorders* (DSM): depression, anxiety disorders, psychoses, substance use disorders, and eating disorders. This background is meant to inform the MHFA action plan called ALGEE: *A*ssess for suicide risk, *L*isten nonjudgmentally, *G*ive reassurance/information, *E*ncourage professional help, and *E*ncourage self-help/support.

Education programs vary in audience. The four types defined by Jorm target the average adult, how to sensitize them to their own mental health service needs as well as loved ones and peers. Other groups, however, are also important targets of mental health education. Programs seek to enhance psychiatric literacy of students and practitioners of mental health disciplines, informing them about the evolving landscape of evidence-based practices as well as service gatekeepers such as primary care physicians or nurse practitioners trained on assessments for early identification. The amount of work in this area is epic.

INFORMATION OVERLOAD

There seems to be never-ending optimism to educational positivism that leads to a ceaseless rush for more and more information. These programs, however, are often muted by information overload. Consider two examples. Primary care providers (PCPs) are recognized as essential partners for engaging people with mental illness in psychiatric care. In this spirit, education programs teach them strategies to identify, among other things, suicide risk, depression, trauma abuse, substance use disorder, and early psychosis (Centers for Disease Control, 2010). PCPs must balance these priorities with related public safety concerns about domestic violence, guns in the house, riding without seat belts, and texting while driving. Along with this is attention to physical health assessment to identify cancer markers, promote healthy lifestyles, and monitor heart health. Addressing these priorities is a righteous goal to be sure, but likely overwhelms PCPs with yet additional tasks to their already busy practice day. By the way, identification is only the first step of the task. The PCPs' work increases exponentially when positive indicators emerge. They must then find available mental health providers to whom the person is referred.

Similarly, consider the overload of MHFA. One of its strengths is reducing knowledge down to action: ALGEE. However, are five of eight MHFA chapters on symptoms and disease necessary as foundation to this action? After all, CPR students do not need to know the pathophysiology of the heart to successfully use its guidelines to check airways and begin chest massage. In addition, effective action plans embedded in educational programs need to be behaviorally simple. Consider, for example, that maintaining respiratory and cardiac functioning rests on simple evaluation, mouth-to-mouth resuscitation, and external cardiac massage. ALGEE lacks behavioral simplicity, in part, because the act of engaging a person in distress and orienting them to seeking help is hugely nuanced.

The impact of information overload varies between onetime education events (e.g., a single seminar for PCPs on assessing suicide risk) and distributed education (e.g., learning to connect evidence-based interventions with corresponding syndromes over repeated training in a yearlong program). Onetime education is restricted by processing capacity in the relatively brief time of training. Program participants in an hour-long session are only able to attend to limited information in the cacophony of a health class. Even less of this information is then encoded into meaningful existing schemas ("What the person already knows about suicide risk."), transferred from short- to long-term memory, subsequently retrieved, and translated to action ("He's suicidal. I need to refer him to the psychiatrist on call."). Capacity in the discrete setting is the lens through which finite and relatively limited information passes. Hence, educators need to select information for their program sparingly, making sure to focus on a simple and brief behavior change goal.

Information overload impacts distributed learning given that ongoing classes occur in the larger sphere of cyberspace (e.g., online sites, social media, e-mail volume, cell phone calls, and devise maintenance) and place-based channels (home and at-work demands and noise; print, television, and radio). Cyber-based information overload is actually associated with more stress and poorer health as well as confusion about appropriate health decision making. Research on cancer information overload leads to information avoidance, the active effort to eschew information channels that might improve knowledge about the course of different cancers and corresponding, evidence-based interventions (Chae, Lee, & Jensen, 2016). Learning is a finite reservoir that permits only so much information to be internalized when distributed over time. New information may not be able to offset what is already in the reservoir. Alternatively, new knowledge might supplant what has already been learned.

Education positivism needs to be tempered. More is not better but might worsen outcomes because of information overload. Three guidelines are useful for educators. (1) Processing capacity is a limited resource not to be wasted. Attempt at mental health literacy may consume capacity that cannot be used elsewhere. Primary care physicians do not need to waste learning time by reviewing the neurophysiology of depression as part of a program to learn screens for suicide risk. MHFA students do not need hours of training on the DSM for program graduates to engage others about mental health challenges. Make sure training programs are anchored by simple and brief behavioral prescriptions.

(2) Know that new training may interfere with already-learned skills. Suicide screens may diminish when primary care providers subsequently

I do not come to education skepticism lightly. I spent years in higher education pursuing multiple degrees. This was the singular focus of my young adult life; because of my mental health challenges, a program that should have taken six years actually required more than a dozen. I tried to balance being a young married man and father with lectures, tests, and papers. I was committed to learning the fundamentals of my profession in coursework and practice. I translated this to being a service provider my first fifteen years post grad school, setting up interventions meant to assist people with psychiatric disabilities attain their life goals. I was director of a program that provided more than twenty thousand patient hours per year while at the University of Chicago. Our program sought to improve life skills of people with mental illness through psychoeducation. I also directed a psychiatric rehabilitation training program for service providers across the state of Illinois. I believed we could advance the needs of people with serious mental illness if service providers better understood psychiatric disability and evidence-based practice.

About twelve years ago, I changed direction deciding to replace my practitioner hat for psychology professor at the Illinois Institute of Technology. I now teach students in courses that provide them with principles and practices that make them better counselors. These are not fleeting relationships. I have doctoral students who study with me for seven or eight years from bachelor's to PhD. That's like going to medical school, twice.

I was an educational positivist. I believed people with lived experience could learn social and problem-solving skills that would help them master their disability. I believed rehabilitation providers could learn program skills that help people master their disability despite social or cognitive dysfunctions. When I changed focus to stigma, I believed public stigma is squelched when the "normal" majority learns the truth about mental illness and recovery.

I've been disappointed by education. Skills training to overcome disabilities is limited, especially when it is removed from the real world in which goals are sought. Program development training is limited by the perspectives and priorities of staff charged with developing and maintaining these programs. Most sobering, education effects on stigma are nearly absent.

Although I write here as a heretic, I am not ready to jettison education. I am not giving up my professorial job nor am I turning away from the potential of education to further strategies that help people achieve their personal goals. However, I have given up educational positivism. I recognize the limits of education and make sure these limits do not prevent me from identifying other ways to promote agenda against stigma and for recovery.

focus on domestic violence. Consider how new behaviors might be intertwined with existing approaches. For example, how might suicide screens be integrated with already existing efforts to identify depression? (3) Take the big picture and ask how specific programs advance literacy across the breadth of community health priorities. A proverbial "master" plan is necessary to make sure good intentions of one group do not interfere with another. Institutions such as schools or professional associations need these plans for an overall curriculum of health pursuits. This is a daunting task because administrators may need to decide to pursue one goal while omitting another.

MESSAGE CHOICES

Despite its limitations, research on education has led to insights about messaging. Slogans that might seem to make sense may worsen stigma and undermine affirming attitudes and actions. Consider, for example, normalcy: "People with mental illness are just like me." Goffman (1963) characterized stigma as "undesired differentness" that results from a mark discrediting an outgroup from the majority. People with mental illness are different from the norm and, hence, somehow broken. One might think accentuating similarities between people with mental illness and the "normal" majority through an appeal to normalcy decreases stigma. Insights from other stigmatized groups suggest, however, that celebrating different-ness may better decrease stigma. Consider American society moving away from a 1960s idea of color-blindness (that all races are the same and, there-fore, should not be stigmatized) to the notion of black power and apprecia-tion of African heritage. In this case, society's goal was to celebrate differentness by promoting acceptance and solidarity.

There are unintended effects to "normalcy" representations; people with mental illness might be expected to keep aspects of their identity secret or to accentuate their normalcy. There are consequences to suppressing aspects of one's identity that harm a person's mental and physical health, relation-ships, and well-being (Smart & Wegner, 2000). Individuals of color and women who identify with their stigmatized group—who proudly tout it publicly—report less stress due to prejudice and better self-esteem (Brans-combe, Schmitt, & Harvey, 1999). The issue of public identity for lesbian, gay, bisexual, transgender, questioning (LGBTQ) persons is a bit more complicated because they need to publicly disclose their orientation. Despite the risks, coming out has generally been found to improve mental and phys-ical health (Beals, Peplau, & Gable, 2009).

Identity and disclosure may have positive or negative aspects on people with mental illness. Those with psychiatric illness may identify with their illness and describe themselves negatively in terms of their distress, failures, or symptoms. They might try to alter this kind of self-image in psychotherapy, spiritual endeavors, or related activity. Mental illness identity, however, can also be viewed positively, leading to a sense of pride. People experience pride in achieving a standard recognized by their culture (e.g., a medal for the runner) or set by themselves (e.g., a personal best race time). Overcoming challenges of mental illness, withstanding related societal stigma, and dem-onstrating a sense of resilience may lead to identity pride. "I did it. I got through college despite having been hospitalized for schizophrenia!" But, pride viewed this way has risk that unintentionally reflects the medical view of recovery, namely, that pride is only achieved when symptoms are remitted and disabilities resolved. What happens to the person who does not experi-ence such outcomes? Pride also comes to people with mental illness as they attain some sense of agency over their lives. Despite recurring psychoses, the person with schizophrenia is able to identify goals worth pursuing and achievable with reasonable accommodations.

Pride also emerges from a sense of who one is; ethnic pride is an example. "I am Irish American" does not suggest any accomplishment per se but rather an additional answer to the person's search to understanding, "Who am I?" I did nothing to earn this identity but every March 17 I proudly fly my Irish colors. In this light, mental illness may be an identity in which some individuals might be proud—the recognition that "I am a person with mental illness" defines much of their daily experience. This kind of identity promotes authenticity and recognition of one's internal conceptualizations in the face of an imposing world.

What then becomes the goal of stigma change programs? The "normal" majority needs to acknowledge positive aspects of some people's identity with mental illness and do this by standing in solidarity with them. Solidarity has two meanings here. First, people with stigmatized conditions gain strength through association with peers—solidarity in a segment of the world. More broadly, however, is the experience where the majority stands with the group who is publicly out with their stigmatized identity, where they say they are in solidarity with people in recovery. The message changes from this perspective. Instead of "Normalcy: although you have a mental illness, you are in most ways just like me," the message becomes "Solidarity: because of your experiences with mental illness, you are a different, respected person. I stand with you." The gay community has definitely embraced solidarity. Once, society might have urged the lesbian to pass as normal, as a straight woman, in order to avoid the harm of homophobia. But the LGBTQ community, and its allies, clearly recognize now that embracing who one is, including one's sexual orientation, is essential to well-being. Instead of passing, the gay community expects the rest of the world to stand with them.

PARITY NOT PITY

People are motivated by pity to help those who are sick. They are moved to remedy painful symptoms and significant challenges that undermine hope, achievement, and well-being. Illness moves others to sympathy, especially for those who answer the call of health care vocations. Stigma adds to the harm of health challenges. Not only do people have to cope with symptoms and disabilities but they must deal with unfair beliefs and discriminatory reactions against them evoking even greater sympathy. Pity motivates advocates who seek to tear down the stigma of health conditions.

Is pity a good motivator for anti-stigma interventions and research? Bernard Weiner (1995) viewed pity as a mediator between attributions about a condition or event and subsequent help. Those in the "normal" majority who perceive sick patients as *victims* of external agents (e.g., cancer is genetic and not by choice) are likely to be pitied; others will reach out and help the pitied person. Hence, public service campaigns focus on the need for more resources to help innocent patients get the treatment they need. Although perhaps well intentioned, this reflects a dated notion of charity; namely, that those with resources (the healthy and the provider) should *bestow* on others (the sick) advantages held by the first. Charity exacerbates the power hierarchy between those with illness and their healthy family, friends, and health care providers. With stigma also comes loss of power. Pity exacerbates power loss. In the guise of concern and intention, pity flames notions that sick people are somehow less than everyone else. Peter Byrne from University College, London, once taught me what people with lived experience seek—not pity but parity. They don't want a leg up. They want the opportunities that everyone deserves.

The pity narrative is seductive. In the media we know "if it bleeds, it leads." Most progressives would likely object to using tawdry stories of violence (Addict kills three in drug induced frenzy!) and sex (Stripper gets HIV in Boys Town!) to promote health agendas. But pity is used in this light; pictures and stories of the untreated illness make for compelling front pages, especially examples of worst rather than typical outcomes. Advocates are likely to use stories of failed health in order to attract donors and foundations to their causes. Children in those stories are especially potent draws. Although we may win pyrrhic victories, the more insidious message remains. People with illness are less than us, different from us. Difference is the base on which stigma rests.

While being wary of pity, we should not deny that some people are victimized by illness and the stigma that creates it. Nor should we turn away from those misfortunes and injustices. But, we must also be alert to reifying victimhood by making people victims, by teaching them that "wounded" is now part of their identity. This kind of equation has been shown to undermine the person's search for individual dignity (Meredith, 2009).

CONTINUITY NOT CATEGORY

The sense of differentness that flames stigma is worsened by categorical conceptualizations of mental illness, that people labeled with psychiatric disorders are somehow in a class that is qualitatively distinct from the norm. Diagnostic labels do this. Instead of being a person, the individual is now branded with schizophrenia. Advocates have proposed continuum beliefs as an alternative to the categorical messages of biogenetic explanations. In continuum beliefs, symptoms and disabilities of mental illness are framed as differences on a scale of behavior rather than as qualitatively distinct phenomena. Visual hallucinations, for example, vary along a continuum from the most pathognomonic (clearly seeing people who are not there), to vague images (glowing auras), to corner-of-the-eye experiences ("Was that my dead Aunt Gertrude I just saw?"), to "normal" vision. Framing symptoms such as visual hallucinations on a continuum reduces stigma by decreasing categorical beliefs about those with serious mental illness and everyone else. In fact, those in the "normal" majority who endorse continuum beliefs are less likely to endorse social distance.

The Hearing Voices Movement (HVM) is a radical extension of this idea. Established by Romme and Escher in the 1980s, the HVM rests on a fundamental quarrel with the medical model (Escher & Romme, 2012). Instead of viewing auditory hallucinations as pathognomonic of psychoses—and therefore as irrefutable evidence for psychiatric intervention including medication—the HVM views voices as another quality of human diversity. Many people experience voices without being symptomatic. The HVM believes Western medicine bastardized historical comprehension of voices from spiritual and valued to sick and diminished over thousands of years of cultural development (Johnson, 1978). HVM replaces pathological models with a three-phase model of recovery.

1. Startling: First experiences with voices are strange and alarming.
2. Organization: People make sense of their voices and learn to accept them. This may include coping strategies that help them better manage the stress that often accompanies voices.

3. Stabilization: Over time, people establish a sense of equilibrium and accommodation that allows them to continue their journey of hope and self-determination.

The HVM includes a peer-led safe space for individuals to share their experiences without risk of pathologizing responses. The program is especially popular in the United Kingdom with more than 200 active groups.

EDUCATING CHILDREN

Education programs may have benefits for children because their cognitive abilities are less developed than adults' abilities are. As a result, children are often viewed as important targets for stigma change; perhaps preschool and primary grade children could be influenced such that prejudice about and discrimination toward people with mental illness never develops or is muted. We might foster future generations where the stigma of mental illness is neither so prevalent nor egregious. These kinds of programs require better understanding of how stigma develops and is maintained in children. I contrast two cognitive models that explain prejudice and stereotype development—incremental learning and cognitive stage models—that have been used to explain the stigma experience of children related to ethnicity. Summaries of the research are complex but lead to some intriguing generalizations. I extrapolate these ideas to mental illness stigma and stigma change.

Research on ethnic stigma suggests that children as young as three are sensitive to cues that signal group differences and hence may be born with these preferences. Children at this age are able to discriminate between black and white, assign racial labels, and identify to which groups they belong (Aboud, 1988; Augoustinos & Rosewarne, 2001). Children seem to be born with the capacity to cognitively differentiate and segregate. Interestingly, children are able to perform these perceptual tasks without being aware of the racial concepts, classifications, or stereotypes that accompany them. By five years of age, children are knowledgeable about and can report outgroup stereotypes (Aboud, 2003). They also report that they personally believe them. Interestingly, knowing stereotypes does not lead to agreeing with them. Seven-year-olds show the same level of stereotype about people of color but lower levels of prejudice. In particular, a marked decrease in prejudice toward people of color is noted as children age from five to seven. This improvement seems to represent less prejudicial beliefs about the out-group rather than less favoritism towards the in-group.

Do learning stereotypes, yielding prejudice, and behaving in discrimi-natory ways develop in a progressive incremental fashion or in qualitative leaps signifying discrete cognitive stages? Classic social psychological the-ory supports the former model; namely, children are born with no stereo-types, prejudice, and/or discrimination and slowly acquire them through interactions with parents, peers, and other key people in the child's life (Stephan, 1999). The incremental model, however, has not been supported by research in two ways. First, a significant association between parent and young child attitudes should be found. It has not (Aboud & Doyle, 1996).

Second, younger children should typically show lower scores on measures of the constructs than older children because prejudice and discrimination are acquired incrementally. Children a few years younger than seven fre-quently endorse negative statements about out-groups at a higher rate than older children. Proponents of the incremental learning model have an answer for this finding. As children age from five to seven, they learn social desirability rules that teach them to constrain their prejudicial beliefs (Katz, Sohn, & Zalk, 1975). For example, parents teach their children to suppress prejudicial statements in order to avoid social opprobrium. Alter-natively, change from high to low prejudice, as a child ages from five to seven, is often used as evidence that supports the cognitive stage model of prejudice development.

COGNITIVE STAGES

A stage model represents classic developmental theory of Piaget (1985) and its more contemporary manifestations (Flavell, 1999). According to these models, children cognitively develop through a series of stages during which qualitatively distinct abilities emerge. Piaget, for example, grouped children into sensorimotor (birth to three years old), preoperational (three to five years old), and concrete operational stages (older than seven). Children toward the end of the sensorimotor stage have acquired the ability to perceive their world, though they have limited skills for putting these perceptions to language. Their perceptions are largely egocentric and limited to one aspect of a situation at a time. Three-year-old children who have completed the sensorimotor stage of cognitive development are perceptually able to distinguish cues that distinguish in-groups from out-groups and identify with their in-group. Language abilities are limited so they are unable to voice stereotypes that correspond with in-group–out-group distinctions. Preoperational five-year-olds have acquired sufficient language abilities so they are able to recount stereotypes that correspond with these differences distinctions. Knowledge of stereotypes markedly increases. The five-year-old's inability to avail complex cognitive processes and their overall egocentrism prevents them from separating knowledge of stereotypes from personally believing them. Dominated by one dimension of appraisal, the unsophisticated preoperational child may conclude that the in-group is good and the out-group is bad (Aboud, 2003). Hence, they appear to endorse prejudicial statements about stigmatized groups.

Expanded conceptual abilities of individuals in the concrete operational stage explain the noticeable reduction in prejudice from age five to seven. For example, research has shown that white children with higher test scores on multiple classification measures were less likely to endorse racial prejudice regardless of age (Aboud, 2003). This pattern explains the dip in prejudice as children age beyond five years.

There are important differences between ethnic and psychiatric outgroups that need to be considered when extrapolating these findings to the stigma of mental illness. First, cues that signal stigmatizing reactions to people of color are relatively manifest while those leading to prejudice against people with mental illness are hidden. The prejudice related to ethnicity seen at a young age (three to five years) is attributed to perception of difference in skin color and the relatively unsophisticated attribution that emerges from preoperational children—that *different* is bad. We would expect same age children are unable to perceive cues that distinguish people with mental illness from the "normal" population; as a result, they will be less likely to endorse prejudicial statements about this group at age five. This hypothesis is supported by data that show seven-year-olds were unfamiliar and confused by terms like *mental illness* and *psychiatry* (Spitzer & Cameron, 1995). Prejudice against those with mental illness occurs as the result of more mature, concrete, operational cognitive abilities as the child ages when they are able to perceive outgroup differences in people with mental illness.

Second, comprehension of outgroup identity and status for people with mental illness is distinct between people of color and individuals with serious mental illness. In terms of ethnicity, we assume, for example, that African American children view blacks as the in-group and whites as the out-group. The unique characteristics of different ethnic groups are essential for intergroup perceptions. This kind of assumption does not explain groupness in mental illness. The "normal" group exists only in juxtaposition to the group of people with psychiatric symptoms. Consider the point conversely; the concept of normal groupness makes no sense without a prior group of people labeled as abnormal.

Research on ethnic prejudice suggests that as children move from age five to seven years old, prejudice decreases because attributions about outgroups moderate (Aboud, 1988). Namely, negative statements of seven-year-olds are moderated by more positive statements about the ethnic out-group. How might this moderation appear in mental illness given the traditional differentiation of in-groups and out-groups used to describe ethnic groups may not apply? Put another way, are there any positive attributes about the mental illness group that can be perceived as children cognitively mature? Positive beliefs/experiences about African Americans included highly supportive extended family, strong religious orientation, and acceptance of gender equity. Negative beliefs/experiences included stereotypes about dangerousness, lack of ambition, and intelligence. People with mental illness identified a similar slew of negative experiences: stereotypes about dangerousness, incompetence, unpredictability, and childishness come to mind. However, positive experiences or beliefs about mental illness were more difficult to list. Hence, as children age, they may report fewer negative attributes about people with mental illness but show no change in positive attributes about the group per se.

Naively, the reader might think mental illness is a group to which no one strives to be identified. The number one goal is to get out of the group through treatment. Stop the symptoms and the person no longer needs to be in the stigmatized group. However, the peer advocacy of the past fifty years has identified people who identify with the group known publicly as "mentally ill" (Chamberlin, 1978; Deegan, 1990). They have come together for mutual support to battle a frequently hostile mental health system. Their groups have embraced such values as the artistic, spiritual, and communal as a result of their roots in the mental illness group. These positive elements moderate negative stereotypes about people with mental illness for those aware of these values.

STIGMA CHANGE IN CHILDREN

Unfortunately, studies on educational strategies to moderate stigma in children are far fewer than for adults, largely because research protections for children are more restrictive than for adults. People under eighteen must have parental consent to participate in research, a formidable goal in science. What little research that does exist was done on high school and college students or adults. Lessons, however, can be learned from school-based strategies to reduce racism. One review found that 46 percent of schools have some kind of multicultural education program in place (Washburn, Brown, & Robert, 1996). These programs offer knowledge about the historical and cultural contributions of ethnic groups; educators assume that prejudice will diminish as children acquire a more complex picture of the group. Realizing that knowledge is not enough—that relaying objective facts without a sense of importance or empathy will not affect prejudice— researchers have sought to augment education by influencing children's norms about social groups. One common way to influence norms within educational programs is for authorities (e.g., children's teachers) to endorse the antibias message implicit within an education program. These authorities explicitly state that integrated and free interactions among children of all groups are ideal. Minor reductions in racist attitudes of children have been found in this approach (Derman-Sparks & Phillips, 1997; McGregor, 1993). Applying this approach to mental illness stigma, children would be educated about peers with mental illness and teachers would endorse the need for free and fully integrated interactions among children with and without behavioral health challenges.

TRAINING SOCIAL SKILLS

Discrimination against children with mental illness may result because class-mates and friends lack social skills to engage them. Developmental psychologists have taught four- to seven-year-olds social cognitive skills to suppress prejudice. Children at this age have relatively simple concepts of social out-groups; for example, they perceive out-group members as all alike. Strengthening a child's ability to differentiate among members of an out-group reduces prejudice. One way to do this is through a perceptual differentiation task where children are trained to give pictures of several out-group members distinct names thereby increasing the differentiation of the group (Aboud & Fenwick, 1999; Katz & Zalk, 1978). Key element of these tasks is instruction on "variety," which helps the child better perceive differentiation.

ROLE-PLAYING AND EMPATHY

Role-playing strategies that facilitate empathy for outgroup members augment social skills training (Aboud & Levy, 2000). First, role-playing focuses on capabilities that are considered relevant for diminishing the prejudice that impedes intergroup relations. Second, role-playing strategies focus on skills that vary developmentally and can be potentially enhanced by situational exercises. The success of role-playing rests on assumptions that pre-schoolers and kindergarteners are egocentric (unable to assume the perspective of someone different from themselves) and sociocentric (cannot assume the perspective of someone from a different group). Hence, role-playing strategies put children in the other's shoes by instructing them to play the role of out-group peer. Through this kind of acting, children gain perspective of and empathy for the out-group.

PROTEST AND CONSEQUENCES

Protest highlights the injustice of specific stigmas and leads to a moral appeal for people to stop thinking that way—"shame on you for holding such disrespectful ideas!" Although this kind of attitude suppression may yield a rebound effect, protest may be effective as a punishing consequence to discriminatory behavior that decreases odds that people will repeat this behavior. For example, courts ordering punitive damages to be paid by employers who discriminate in hiring is likely to discourage future behavior like this. This example reduces discrimination in adults. An important question for children would be the impact of punishment from authority figures like parents and teachers when the child obviously acts in a discriminatory manner. For example, what is the effect of admonishing a child for acting in a discriminatory manner? "Shame on you Sarah. You should not exclude Betty from the lunch table because she is hyperactive." Generally, punishing contingencies for children (or, for that matter, adults) has unintended consequences. While punishment suppresses behavior soon after the painful consequence, effects of negative consequences often do not maintain. It teaches children what *not* to do. Like behavior change programs in general, strategies to reduce discrimination should include reinforcers to affirmative actions that replace stigma with ideas of recovery. This might, for example, include some privilege from the teacher for participating in an anti-stigma program.

DO NOT FORGET THE PARENTS

Beliefs of children are significantly impacted by parents and other significant adults. Parents who explicitly endorse prejudice and discriminate against people with mental illness are likely to hand these biases down to their children. Hence, programs that seek to change children's attitudes and behaviors need to assess parents' and guardians' thoughts about these beliefs and actions. Parents may need to be included in anti-stigma programs when they endorse bigoted views. This is a formidable challenge especially for programs based in schools. How are parents, absent from school, engaged in anti-stigma programs?

Parental influence on children changes as the child ages. Teenagers, for example, are more likely to reject parental opinion than embrace it. Other important people in the adolescent's network need to be included instead; e.g., friends, coaches, and faith-based community leaders.

SELF-STIGMA AND EDUCATION

Education programs have been developed to impact the self-stigma of mental illness. Content may include didactic review of the myths of mental illness and how internalization of these myths may undermine a person's journey to recovery. These programs, however, are rarely limited to the kind of didactic strategies that define educational programs for the public. Self-stigma has alternatively been understood as maladaptive self-statements that developed through social development where a person first learns mental illness prejudice and internalizes it when they are labeled. Interpersonal differences in cognitive schemata may help explain why, given the same social situation, one person feels significantly "stigmatized," while a second may not feel stigmatized, and a third is motivated to act against it. The adverse effects of stigma are "located" not only in the social situation but in the cognitive process of the stigmatized individual, i.e., the way an individual perceives and understands the social situation such that disrespectful messages emerge.

Aaron Beck's cognitive therapy has been shown to be an effective strategy for helping people change self-statements that cause anxiety, depression, and the consequences of self-stigma. The counselor helps the client explore distressing thoughts, attempting to reframe them as belief rather than fact, empathically discussing how one might arrive at such beliefs (but also recognizing their emotional costs), reviewing evidence for and against the beliefs, and trying to find less-distressing alternative interpretations. Advocates and researchers have adapted cognitive therapy to address self-stigmatizing statements (Yanos, Lucksted, Drapalski, Roe, & Lysaker, 2015). The counselor and client together seek to identify stigmatizing self-statements (I'm weak because I have to take antidepressants.) and then, through collaborative empiricism, work together to "disprove" the stigma (Wait a minute; a lot of successful people take medication.) and replace it with an affirming reframe (I'm not weak because of my medication. I'm smart. It's a big step towards recovery.).

A new approach to cognitive therapy called Acceptance and Commitment Therapy (ACT) has also been adapted for addressing self-stigma (Hayes, Strosahl, & Wilson, 1999). Rather than teaching people to challenge their thoughts, ACT educates individuals to be mindful of self-stigma and accept it. ACT has more of a feeling of Eastern philosophy than Western logic. The harmful effects of internalized self-stigma come less from the thoughts per se and more from their function. Research has shown ACT to have positive effects of changing the stigma of mental illness (Masuda et al., 2007).

THE PARADOX OF FIXING SELF-STIGMA

Focusing on self-stigma may frame the prejudice and discrimination that results as a problem solely of people with mental illness (Corrigan & Fong, 2014). Like the disabilities that arise from their illness, stigma is another unfortunate result of having mental illness with which people inflicted with the disease must learn to live. This kind of perspective ignores the responsibility that the "normal" majority has in creating and maintaining stigma. Although there is value in consumers of mental health services and others victimized by stigma learning how to deal with its harm, it should not release the "normal" majority from its responsibility. Bruce Link and colleagues (1991) argued that because stigma is powerfully reinforced by culture, its effects are not easily overcome by the coping actions of individuals. Labeling and stigma are "social problems" that need to be addressed by public approaches not "individual troubles" that are addressed by personal/private therapies. Although this view risks being one-sided in limiting itself to interventions aimed only at the society at large (research supports the conclusion that both individual-level and society-level interventions can be useful), it is true that the self-stigma experienced by some people with mental illness is less likely to thrive if the "normal" majority, as a whole, refuses to nurture stereotypes, prejudice, and discrimination.

Self-stigma steals power. People with a strong sense of personal empowerment have higher self-efficacy and self-esteem. Rather than being overwhelmed by symptoms and labels, empowered people have a positive outlook and take an active role in their recovery. Hence, strategies that promote empowerment may have significant effects on self-stigma. Communities and health service providers can foster personal empowerment among mental health clients in a variety of ways that involve giving consumers greater control over their own treatment and integration into the community. This begins by including the person in all facets of intervention that help attain vocational and independent-living goals.

7

BEATING STIGMA PERSON
TO PERSON

P ERSON-TO-PERSON CONTACT HAS long been recognized as an effective
means for reducing prejudice between groups. Consider how attitudes
changed about the lesbian, gay, bisexual, transgender, questioning
(LGBTQ) community. It was not because people *learned* that sexual orientation was genetic and hence did not choose to be gay. It was not because
our children learned in health class about heredity that erased beliefs of
moral responsibility. Attitudes did not improve because they were corrected
by scientific fact. Attitudes changed because straight and gay communities
interacted. They exchanged their aspirations and goals, in the process noting similarities that outranked differences. They met as equals. Contact
helps the straight community to check out stereotypes for themselves, that
gay men are not perverts seeking to prey on children, or gay women are
not butches seeking to be tough guys. The LGBTQ community is as
diverse as the world as a whole. But contact does more than just erase the
negative. Contact promotes the positive where the straight community
experiences the depth and breadth of values and heritage among the gay
community. Together, this kind of contact replaces prejudice and discrimination with affirming attitudes and behaviors.

Gordon Allport (1954), often considered one of the founding fathers of
social psychology, identified four elements of effective contact: (1) *Equal status between groups*. In the contact situation, neither the figure nor the
ground occupies higher status. Both people with mental illness and the

"normal" majority interact as peers. This differs from the type of contact certain power groups typically have with persons with mental illness (e.g., landlord/resident, employer/employee, doctor/patient). (2) *Common goals.* Both groups should be working toward similar ends. Some approaches to contact have used contrived tasks such as working jointly on a puzzle. Contact, however, is more powerful when the two groups work together on a community project or solving a neighborhood problem. For example, members of a mosque that include individuals of the congregation with mental illness and "normal" majority could join forces to offer a weekly meal to people who are homeless in the area, many who might be challenged by serious mental illness. (3) *No competition.* The tone of the contact should be a joint effort, not a competitive one. Obviously, the normal ground is not gathered in contact exercises to argue against the rights of those with mental illness. But equally important, those with mental illness should seek full belonging without hostile messages about bigoted normals. (4) *Authoritative sanction for the contact.* Specific interventions are sponsored or endorsed by management of an employment organization or by particular community organizations (e.g., the board of education or the Better Business Bureau). Contact in a synagogue will only be effective if the rabbi proudly and prominently introduces the person with mental illness to the congregation from the pulpit: "here is a fellow human being with an important message, one which I hope we all heed."

Some contacts seem to be better than others. Individuals that highly disconfirm prevailing stereotypes may not be believed as representative, instead being viewed as "special exceptions." The "normal" majority may not believe an award-winning celebrity has a mental illness, especially for first contact. This is why famous people coming out have limited effects on changing public attitudes. Demi Lovato has disclosed challenges due to eating disorders, Britney Spears due to bipolar disorder, and Mel Gibson with bipolar disorder. Star power brings needed light to concerns about stigma. But its effect on lasting change is limited by what I call the Thurgood Marshall effect. Justice Marshall was the first African American on the U.S. Supreme Court, appointed by President Johnson in 1967. Many progressives hoped that having Justice Marshall on the bench would change prejudice about America's black community, thinking "he's a distinguished and able individual so most African Americans must be too."

Unfortunately, it does not work that way. White people compartmentalize knowledge about Justice Marshall. He's not like most black people. And so the "normal" majority does the same thing. Famous people with mental illness are not like most people with mental illness. This may explain the limited effect of *Beautiful Mind*, the biopic about Nobel laureate John Nash, on stigma change. Nash's accomplishments do not generalize to more positive expectations about people with schizophrenia because he is not like most people with serious mental illness.

Conversely, contact with persons who behave in ways consistent with stereotypes about their group may reinforce stigmatizing attitudes. Meeting a disheveled man on the street who is shouting at his voices does not decrease stigma. If anything, it makes it worse. This may be one reason why psychiatrists and psychologists are consistently among the most stigmatizing of professionals. Providers see people with mental illness mostly when they are acutely ill where exchanges largely reinforce stereotypes about people with mental illness being overwhelmed by symptoms and out of control.

Moderate disconfirmation works best. This is the person who has struggled with serious psychiatric symptoms, been engaged in care, and achieved some semblance of recovery. This person has achieved personal goals including a satisfying vocation and living independently. Contact is most effective when bridging relationships between the "normal" majority and their coworkers, neighbors, fellow church goers, relatives, and friends, all with mental illness. Ironically, these relationships always existed. Contact removes the secrecy so members of the "normal" majority can discover these relationships for themselves. Discovery is an especially potent aspect of the power of contact.

THE EFFECTIVE MESSAGE

Effective messages for people seeking to moderately disconfirm stereotypes include three components: on-the-way-down story, on-the-way-up rejoinder, and change moral. On-the-way-down stories summarize personal challenges of mental illness and interventions. The story shares what it is like to, for example, hear voices, be unable to think clearly, be overwhelmed by sadness, or consider suicide. Sometimes it seems that the person with mental illness needs to "qualify" as a real person with mental illness. Rarely would an audience dismiss a man's story as being gay. "You say you're gay, I believe you're gay." Not always so for mental illness. Often the "normal" majority does not believe someone who presents well could have ever been the kind of patient who was in the hospital, messy, and unable to get out of bed. The person needs to qualify to prove they have a serious mental illness. This happens by sharing diagnostic labels, psychiatric care, medications, and hospitalization.

Sometimes stories err by only focusing on-the-way-down. This is the emotionally compelling part of the person's journey, the blood and guts for the audience. Speakers and audience alike are drawn to it. On-the-way-down is the foreign experience of symptoms and treatment seen on hospital wards, with forced treatment and Nurse Ratched. Erasing stigma, however, only occurs after the on-the-way-up rejoinder! On-the-way-up is the story of "despite." Despite symptoms and disabilities, the person has achieved. The person has aspirations like everyone and took the steps necessary to accomplish them. Achievement, by the way, is not measured by some external standard of college education, six-figure income, home in the suburbs, or multiple children. Ethicists would never presume that someone who works in a Walmart and lives in a one-bedroom apartment in the city has somehow not achieved. The anti-stigma story is cast in the same light. Everyone can achieve goals.

The story ends with a three-part moral:

1. My story is real, not the exception. People recover, even those with schizophrenia who have been hospitalized several times.

2. Despite my achievements, I experience stigma. The prejudice and discrimination that results from my label has robbed me of opportunities. It has forced me into a closet where I unjustly feel ashamed of myself. Stigma can be as big a hurdle to recovery as the mental illness itself.

3. Hence, stigma has to be stopped and affirming attitudes have to be promoted. This is an issue of society-wide injustice. Just as progressive communities no longer tolerate racism, sexism, and homophobia, so communities must own programs meant to erase the stigma of mental illness.

Sometimes after telling my story, someone will respond, "For real. Are you really mentally ill? You look too good to have ever been a mental patient!" That is why I have developed a story that meets the implicit criteria for truly being mentally ill.

- I have a label. I have alternately been diagnosed with bipolar disorder, major depression, and anxiety disorder with panic.
- It has been going on for a long time. I have struggled with my illness on and off for more than forty years.
- It has derailed my life. I dropped out of medical school, grad school at the University of Chicago, UCLA postdoc, and faculty position at Northwestern University.
- I have needed some serious treatment.
  - □ I have been seen by psychiatrists for more than twenty-five years.
  - □ I have had to rush to emergency clinics.
  - □ I have been hospitalized for my mental illness.
  - □ I have taken psychiatric medications, sometimes with major side effects.

When I first started telling my story, I was embarrassed by some of this and left it out. But as my story developed, it evolved to include all these points so the audience knew, "Yep. I've had the REAL mental illness that led to some major disabilities."

RESEARCH EVIDENCE

How does contact compare to the other major form of anti-stigma program, education? One review summarized seventy-nine studies, thirteen of which were of the most rigorous form, randomized controlled trials. Results showed adults who participated in contact had significantly better changes in stigmatizing attitudes and behavioral intentions than those who participated in education alone (Corrigan, Morris, Michaels, Rafacz, & Rusch, 2012). Benefits for contact were two to three times greater than for education. A subsequent analysis suggests benefits of contact were maintained better over time than those of education (Corrigan, Michaels, & Morris, 2015).

STRATEGIC STIGMA CHANGE

Strategic Stigma Change (SSC) are guidelines that summarize the most effective approach to stigma change and are defined by the acronym TLC4: Targeted, Local, Credible, Continuous, CONTACT leading to Change. SSC rests on person-to-person contact. Effective change only occurs when led by the person with lived experience. Contact is enhanced by five other actions.

1. CONTACT NEEDS TO BE TARGETED

Rather than focusing on the population as a whole, contact is more effective when it targets key groups, especially people in positions of power such as employers, landlords, and health care providers. They hold the keys to opportunity related to work, independent living, health, and wellness. Other important target groups include faith-based and community leaders, legislators, school personnel, entitlement counselors, and media outlets. Venue and timing are key considerations in targeted contact. Where, for example, are good places to contact targets? Large numbers of employers can be contacted through civic groups such as Rotary International or the Optimist Club. Civic groups are places where leaders have made commitments to improve their community by virtue of group membership. Times and opportunities for planned contacts may already exist. For example, weekly staff meetings and medical grand rounds offer excellent opportunities for contacting health care providers. All elements that define the target inform the message. On-the-way-down stories review illness and disabilities. Despite this, the person has been able to meet work credentials, get a job, and work it well: on-the-way-up. Moral: people with mental illness are able to be good employees. Hire them with reasonable accommodations.

2. LOCAL CONTACT PROGRAMS ARE MORE EFFECTIVE

The interests of target groups are influenced by locally defined priorities. "Local" has several meanings including geopolitical and diversity factors. It is reasonable to assume, for example, that a target group's interests are shared within a geographical region, such as the Northeast, or more narrowly within a state, such as Vermont. Nevertheless, Vermont is more homogeneous than other states with greater variation in rural, urban, and suburban considerations. It is also important to consider sociopolitical factors in more narrowly defined areas. Large cities include neighborhoods of varying socioeconomic status, and this variation is likely to influence target group interests. For example, employers in impoverished parts of a city and in wealthy suburbs will require different types of contact. Resources for people with mental illness differ in rural and urban areas, which call for different contact programs. Research findings on racial-ethnic disparities in health and health care underline the importance of considering ethnicity and religious background in crafting local contact programs.

3. CONTACTS MUST BE CREDIBLE

Three considerations guide credibility. First, the contact should embody the targeted audience; that is, the individual in the contact role should be similar in ethnicity, religion, and socioeconomic status to the target group. Second, the contact should be in a role similar to that of the target group. Ideally, employers, landlords, health care providers, and police officers who have mental illness should make a presentation to other employers, landlords, health care providers, and police officers. Although appealing, this approach has problems. People in certain roles who publicly disclose their mental illness may experience serious consequences; for example, police officers in some jurisdictions may lose their gun permit, thereby ending their law enforcement career. Alternatively, people from the targeted group might accompany individuals telling their story. For example, employers should tell other employers that a person in recovery will be a good worker. This leads to a contact partnership, which combines a person with lived experience as the contact with target group member (an employer) who speaks familiarly to the "normal" majority (other employers). A compelling Rotary meeting would feature a person with mental illness who talks about her recovery, followed by a presentation from her boss, who describes the successes that resulted from hiring her.

The third consideration—that the person with lived experience should be in recovery—is a bit more complex. Interactions are most effective with

I first introduced TLC4 at a World Psychiatric Association meeting on stigma convened in Ottawa, Canada. The importance of "local" became clear. American ideas have little value in Canada. Things weren't much better when returning home. I am from Chicago in America's heartland. Midwesterners believe everyone on the East Coast is zoned out on caffeine and on the West Coast spaced out on marijuana. Midwesterners have their own vision. Illinois is far from homogeneous. Although the Chicago area is about half of Illinois' population, the rest is largely farms and small towns. Downstaters view Chicagoans with more suspicion than Canadians do Yanks. Peoria is right in the middle of the state. "Does it play in Peoria?" nicely sums up the "local" in TLC4. Do citizens from the Peoria area agree an anti-stigma program represents not only their interests but their approach to change?

people with serious mental illnesses who work, live independently, have good relationships, and have a satisfactory quality of life, which are all benchmarks of recovery. However, as discussed in chapter 1, recovery is an elusive concept without clear criteria. For example, recovery is achieved by some people before going back to work or living independently. This view is consistent with the more preferred definition of recovery, a "journey" marked by hope and goal attainment regardless of symptoms. In addition, limiting contacts to people who are "symptom free" may increase public stigma by implying that others with mental illness are somehow less than whole. People in the process of recovery are good contacts for stigma change.

4. CONTACT MUST BE CONTINUOUS

One-time contact may have some positive effects, but effects are likely to be fleeting. Multiple contacts should occur, with the quality of the contact varying over time. "Carbon copies" have limited effects. Having contact with the same person has muted effects. This calls for different peer and target partners and an array of messages, venues, and opportunities. This principle reminds advocates that stigma change is not easily accomplished and requires ongoing efforts with continuous quality assessment of those efforts.

5. EFFECTIVE CONTACT LEADS TO CHANGE

This is another version of the behavior change standard necessary for education programs. Namely, contact programs need to produce discrete change in the audience. Targeting not only suggests the "who" of strategic contact but also the "what"—what needs to be changed. Negative behaviors need to convert to affirming behaviors: more employer hires, landlord leases, and high-quality health services for people with mental illness. Each of these goals involves specific behaviors that are included in anti-stigma objectives. For example, employers with job openings need to interview people with mental illness, consider reasonable accommodations, offer positions, and provide appropriate supervision that may include job coach participation.

There are existing programs that incorporate TLC4 principles. The National Alliance on Mental Illness (NAMI) developed *In Our Own Voice* (IOOV) as an anti-stigma program largely based on contact. It includes five sections:

- **Dark Days:** presenters describe their most difficult experiences with mental illness.
- **Acceptance:** they share how they have come to accept their illness.
- **Treatment:** treatments that helped the person to recover are discussed.
- **Coping Skills:** presenters share their personal set of coping skills.
- **Success, Hopes, and Dreams:** this section conveys recovery and hope as realities.

Research has shown that participation in a group presentation of IOOV compared to control groups led to significantly less social avoidance and less endorsement of other stigmatizing attitudes (Corrigan et al., 2010).

How does contact work? Twentieth-century media critic Marshall McLuhan said the impact of communication is influenced by message as well as medium in which the message is conveyed. Receiving a message through a television qualitatively alters its impact from print media.

Contact messages need to include on-the-way-up rejoinders to show the public that recovery, hope, and inspiration are a reality for people with serious mental illness. But the face-to-face exchange between people with lived experience and their society lifts these words far beyond their simple statement. Through contact, the public can check for itself the humanity of the person with lived experience. Exchange is an essential component of contact's effect on diminishing stigma. Key to contact is the ability of the public to freely question and share with the person with lived experience. This makes the stigma process spontaneous, leading to flash-bulb insights into experiences of mental illness and of recovery.

THE CHALLENGES OF FACE-TO-FACE CONTACT

Contact embodies a fundamental principle of most programs seeking to promote social justice—grassroots ownership. Findings from the meta-analysis showed grassroots contact is most effective when it is face-to-face (Corrigan, Morris et al., 2012). Video-mediated contact leads to positive changes in stigma and affirming attitudes, though much less than when contact occurs in person. Most likely, the difference is due to the essential element of exchange in contact, namely, that members of the "normal" majority can experience people with lived experience in real time. In the process, they can "check out" their private stereotypes about people labeled with mental illness. Unfortunately, face-to-face contact may be a significant hurdle to public health advocates seeking to diminish stigma. Public service campaigns rely on e-media to spread messages to the population relatively quickly. This seems to undermine face-to-face priorities.

The U.S. Department of Veterans Affairs (VA) sought to use TLC4 principles on an Internet medium through its website, www.MakeThe Connection.net (MTC). I was subject matter expert on the project. MTC targeted the services agenda for stigma change, namely, decrease stigma so veterans become better engaged in VA behavioral health services when needed. MTC is a website where veterans and their families might learn from the stories of peers about behavioral health challenges experienced by ex-military (on-the-way-down) and the promise of evidence-based interventions for recovery (on-the-way-up). Stories end with a similar moral: Veterans with mental illness challenges recover when they engage in evidence-based interventions. Stories are *targeted* through a series of drop-down menus that direct site visitors to report previous service (e.g., army, navy, marines, reserves), gender, era (e.g., WWII through Korean War, Vietnam War, post-Vietnam War era, Desert Storm era), and combat experience. I went to the site and clicked army, male, from the present era (OEF, OIF, OND) with combat experience and was presented a video by Jonathan who had been nine years in the Middle East as part of the Army and then Army National Guard. He tells stories of witnessing a young girl dying because of a roadside explosion and a buddy dying by suicide. "They say soldiers change when they come back . . . Seems like everyone around me changed." Jonathan was withdrawing and overwhelmed with frequent thoughts of suicide. "One day. One of my kids said something . . . that I needed help." This was the impetus for Jonathan to obtain services, first through the VA crisis line. He experienced his counselor more like a coach, just focusing on small things at first. "I started believing in myself." Things got better at work. His family was whole again.

On the same page with Jonathan was Kenny, a solider overwhelmed by posttraumatic stress disorder (PTSD) after multiple Iraqi tours. After VA intervention, Kenny reported being in control of his emotions and a much-improved relationship with his wife and son. There was Ed who lost his leg after an improvised explosive device blast; he said his personal journey in spirituality helped him to overcome anxiety and depression. And Brett, who with his wife's support and VA services, was able to overcome the behavioral health challenges that resulted from his Middle East deployments. Note that these stories were all from male Army. Others popped up from Stephanie, Alysse, Ashley, and Sandra when drop-down menus were coded for a female sailor from the current era.

MTC nicely combines education with contact to promote health literacy. The site distinguishes mental health challenges in three meaningfully different ways:

- Signs and symptoms: the markers of specific mental illnesses such as flashbacks, reckless behavior, trouble sleeping, and irritability;

- Conditions: specific syndromes that these symptoms may represent, including bipolar disorder, PTSD, and adjustment disorder; and
- Life events and experiences: relationships, homelessness, and aging.

MTC included life events and experiences recognizing that behavioral health challenges often arise from specific events and do not necessarily represent a neat set of symptoms. Information overload is less a problem on MTC than the kind of omnibus education program described in the previous chapter. Visitors can browse the site for issues specifically of interest to them and not be sidetracked by conditions that do not peek their interest.

MTC also includes a resources tab that sends visitors to more video-taped stories of veterans who have had successful experiences with counseling, medication, self-help, and peer support. The resources tab also includes a locator button where the site visitor can locate resources for a variety of social needs by zip code. Results include the closest VA services as well as relevant programs that might be found through the Substance Abuse and Mental Health Services (SAMHSA) Behavioral Treatment Services Locator as well as the National Resource Directory.

Although online resources like MTC hold significant promise for advancing the services agenda against stigma, face-to-face strategies are still valuable, especially when addressing rights and self-worth agendas. Large-scale programs have struggled to realize this goal. Canada's *Opening Minds*, for example, built its model on more than seventy-five peer/advocate-based programs distributed across the country's ten provinces and three territories. They provided resources and empowered them to target stigma change in three areas: health services, work, and youth. In this way, a peer program in Saskatchewan develops a strategy that represents local Canadians and sounds different from one for fellow citizens in Toronto. This can be a cumbersome process but still necessary to avail face-to-face contact for rights and self-worth agendas.

CONTACT AND SELF-STIGMA:
IT'S ALL ABOUT THE PEER

Chapter 6 ended by noting that strategies that promote empowerment erase self-stigma. The peer community is central to realizing this goal. Contact with advocates with lived experience is a major remedy for those struggling with self-stigma. Peer support and services are provided by individuals with serious mental illness who are in recovery. Individuals who have shared common experiences may be able to provide better support and safer environments than others who have not had a history of psychiatric treatment. Peer supports and services are, by their very nature, recovery oriented because they engender empowerment based on principles of self-determination. These are the keys to erasing self-stigma.

Persons with mental illness have assembled as peers for support and advocacy for well over 150 years (Corrigan, 2016). In 1845, the Alleged Lunatic's Friend Society was established in England. About the same time, Elizabeth Packard wrote of forced commitment by her husband and founded the Anti-Insane Asylum Society in Illinois. Clifford Beers (1923), who wrote about the abuses he experienced when hospitalized for psychiatric problems in *A Mind That Found Itself*, was instrumental in founding the National Committee for Mental Hygiene, which evolved into Mental Health America (MHA). MHA has been instrumental in promoting peer participation in mental health advocacy, planning, and service delivery. In the 1940s, two members of the staff of Rockland State Hospital outside New York City brought together a group of soon-to-be discharged "patients," hoping their friendships might endure after release from the hospital. Their self-help group called "We Are Not Alone Society" later formed what became Fountain House. Other mutual-help groups such as Recovery, Inc. and GROW have also been active for more than fifty years.

Development of the modern American mental health peer movement occurred in the early 1970s independently of these roots. The movement coincided with the self-help revolution and was fueled by deinstitutionalization policies. Like other marginalized groups, people with serious mental illness began to realize they were being denied basic rights, were discriminated against, and were devalued by society. Consequently, these former patients organized to correct these wrongs, demonstrating that they were not powerless victims. These groups had names like the Insane Liberation Front in Oregon, the Mental Patients' Liberation Project in New York, and the Mental Patients' Liberation Front in Boston. In 1972, the voices of people began to be heard with publications like the *Madness Network News*. The annual Conference on Human Rights and Against Psychiatric Oppression started in 1973. The publication of *On Our Own: Patient-Controlled Alternatives to the Mental Health System* by Judi Chamberlain in 1978 was an important milestone for the movement, as peers read about the self-help movement and the development of peer-operated services in the mainstream press.

Some of these early activists had an antipsychiatry bias because they were angry at a system that they felt had abused and dehumanized them. Hence, some called themselves survivors and formed the National Association of Psychiatric Survivors. Note the significance of their word choice— psychiatric survivors did not survive the illness, they survived the treatment. More radical members formed the Support Coalition International, currently called MindFreedom. Others joined the National Depression and Manic Depression Association (now the Depression and Bipolar Support Alliance). The National Mental Health Consumers' Association represented those with more moderate views and took no formal position on forced treatment. This organization is no longer functioning and some of its members have joined the NAMI Consumer Council (Lefley, 2003).

Peer services and supports have increased greatly over the past several years. Results of a SAMHSA survey suggested there were about 7,500 peer support groups and organizations nationally, with about 3,300 being mutual support groups (primarily providing support), 3,000 self-help organizations (which are education and advocacy groups that evolve from local support groups into a single network, and may sponsor and/or support mutual support groups), and 1,100 peer-led services (included programs, businesses, or services controlled and operated by people who have received mental health services) (Goldstrom et al., 2006). Peer services reported more than 40,000 individuals had attended their last meeting, self-help organizations reported having a membership of more than one million, and peer-led services noted serving more than 530,000 individuals in the past year.

The U.S. Department of Veterans Affairs has identified peer support as central to its psychiatric services. A survey of local recovery coordinators

(LRCs) at two-thirds of the VAs reported on the status of implementing peer support in their settings (Chinman, Salzer, & O'Brien-Mazza, 2012). Seventy percent of LRCs report peer support specialists have been hired to fill VA positions. In terms of hiring, 62 percent reported it to be more difficult than filling nonpeer positions. Support from clinical and administrative leadership facilitated hiring greatly. Over half of LRCs reported that implementation was going well with 96 percent stating peer support has had positive effect on veteran care.

WHAT ARE PEER SERVICES?

Who is a peer? They are people with past history of significant mental illness that caused psychiatric disability. There are no litmus tests or inclusion criteria for "peer": hospitalization, medication, length of illness, social security disability, and work disruption. A person does not have to be hospitalized for mental illness to be in the "peer" group. Instead, people who self-identify as individuals with lived experience with serious mental illness are considered peers. Peers who are hired into service positions are usually in recovery; they are able to achieve important life goals including those related to employment despite their disabilities. Peer services combine emotional with instrumental support that is provided by individuals who come together with the specific intent of bringing about social and personal change. Peer support is mutually beneficial through a reciprocal process of giving and receiving based on principles of respect and shared responsibility. Feelings of rejection, discrimination, frustration, and loneliness are combated through this system of sharing, supporting, and assisting others. Peer support in the traditional sense of self-help groups is voluntary and unpaid. However, peers who deliver support services are financially compensated.

Emotional support is communicating acceptance and approval of peers (Magura et al., 2003; Sells, Davidson, Jewell, Falzer, & Rowe, 2006). It is letting others know that they are cared about, valued, and loved. Emotional support leads to a sense of "universality," learning that others have similar problems and/or circumstances, and "group cohesiveness," perceiving that group members understand and accept each other. *Instrumental support* is having people available who assist peers in meeting resource and psychosocial needs. This includes prosaic delivery of material goods and services as well as informational support that involves advice, guidance, and feedback. Because of the empathic, open, and receptive nature of the peer relationship, peers are sometimes comfortable in exploring problems and concerns in the presence of other peers.

The mutuality or reciprocity of peer relationships may be understood in terms of Reissman's (1965) *help-therapy principle*. Advising, assisting, and emotionally supporting others reinforces one's learning of valued attitudes, skills, and behaviors. Helpers enhance their self-esteem through the social approval and appreciation that they receive from those whom they help. Research has shown that giving help to others improved one's feelings of self-worth and self-efficacy, which suppresses self-stigma (Roberts et al., 1999).

Peer services are not limited to mutual help groups. People with serious mental illness may also benefit from peer-provided rehabilitation services, which promote self-esteem. Unlike self-help groups, the peer relationship here is unidirectional and not mutual. There are three types of services that fall within this domain: peer-operated services, peer partnerships, and peer employees. Peer-operated services are planned, administered, and evaluated by individuals with a mental illness. These services occur within a formal organization that is a freestanding legal entity directed by peers and conforming to values of freedom of choice and peer control. Examples of these services include drop-in centers, crisis services, employment, housing, benefits acquisition, case management, advocacy groups, and crisis services. Peers also provide warm lines that are a telephone support system staffed by peers; warm lines have been found to offer an advantage to the traditional mental health system by alleviating crisis hotlines from being burdened by habitual noncrisis callers (Minth, 2005). Peer-operated services receive financial support from a variety of sources, including government grants, private foundations, and/or fee for service.

Peer partnerships are interventions where individuals with lived experience share responsibility for the service with nonpeers. Administration and governance of the peer service are mutually shared by both peers and nonpeers, though primary control of the service itself is with peers. Peer partnerships are comparable to hybrid self-help groups where professionals may play significant leadership roles (Powell, 1985). The nature of services provided through partnership is no different from those in peer-operated services. Peer-operated services are traditionally nonhierarchical, whereas peer partnerships are structurally less egalitarian.

Peer employees are individuals who self-identify as a person with mental illness and are hired either in a designated peer position or into traditional mental health services. Designated peer positions are in some cases provider extenders such as care coordinating aides or peer specialists, or they may be peer counselors, peer advocates, peer care coordinators, or peer companions. Peers as employees offer several benefits. They have a personal perspective on human service and health systems, successful coping strategies, and engagement. Peer employees are positive role models who instill hope in others that recovery is possible. However, there are also concerns about peers as providers such as boundary issues and dual relationships. Peer employees need to be careful about treating service recipients as friends or violating confidentiality. In addition, professional and paraprofessional providers may have difficulty accepting peers as equal in part because of the prejudice of mental illness. Peer employees may require special accommodations, such as job sharing and additional supports.

THE POWER IN THE PEER

Once again, insights here recapitulate experiences learned from other efforts to resolve the injustice of prejudice and description. Racism is tackled by people of color, sexism by women, ageism by seniors, and homophobia by the LGBTQ community. The stigma of mental illness is beaten by advocates with lived experience. Shame wilts in the light of shared experience. Perhaps different here is the unsaid belief that people with mental illness, unlike blacks, women, or gays, are incapable of being empowered and effective advocates because of their disabilities, a form of stigma in its own right. Hence, peers are an especially resounding signal that changes the public dialogue about mental illness.

IDENTITY AND DISCLOSURE

People need to be out if they are to be peers. They need to share past experiences not only with mental health challenges but also with the prejudice and discrimination that come with it. Peers also need to share stories of empowerment and recovery. This requires two steps. First, people need to identify themselves as individuals with mental illness. Second, they need to disclose this identity. These are complex processes indeed.

Social psychologists have shown that individuals who identify with their stigmatized group report less stress arising from prejudice and better self-esteem. This has been demonstrated for African Americans (Branscome, Schmitt, & Harvey, 1999), older adults (Gartska, Schmitt, Branscome, & Hummert, 2004), women (Schmitt, Branscombe, Kobrynowicz, & Owen, 2002), and the LGBTQ community (Halpin & Allen, 2004). The latter group is especially relevant for understanding the experiences of identity and mental illness because LGBTQ orientation and mental illness are characteristics that are not readily obvious to the public (compared, for example, to skin color for ethnicity or body features for gender). Gays and people with mental illness might deny self-perceptions consistent with a stigmatized role to escape the prejudice and discrimination. For example, people with sexual orientations that differ from the majority might distance themselves from thoughts and behaviors consistent with their orientation to control harmful self-statements (e.g., I am morally weak because I am attracted to people of the same gender). Conversely, LGBTQ persons who accept and hold close their sexual orientation experience not only have less self-stigma but greater self-esteem as well as health and wellness.

Given this, one might think that people with mental illness should identify with that illness. Opinions, however, are mixed. Some support the health value of avoiding a mental illness identity. Research, for example, has found correlations between assuming a "sick patient" role and subsequent pessimism (Lally, 1989). In addition, persons with serious mental illnesses such as schizophrenia may lack a cogent sense of self, including poor insight into the illness. Finally, people who believe identifying with mental illness threatens their broader well-being are likely to suppress that identity (Rüsch et al., 2009a,b). This would seem to imply that identity as a person with mental illness should be avoided.

The relationship between identity and self-stigma is complex, however. Research has shown that effects of illness identity are influenced by perceived legitimacy of mental illness stigma (Lysaker, Davis, Warman, Strasburger, & Beattie, 2007). Those who identified with mental illness but also agree with the stigma of their disorder ("I guess that's right; people with mental illness choose their illness cause they're weak.") report less hope and self-esteem. Conversely, persons whose sense of self prominently included their mental illness and who rejected the stigma of mental illness showed not only more hope and better self-esteem but enhanced social functioning as well. Hence, identifying with mental illness does not automatically lead to more stress; it is the perceived legitimacy of the stigma that threatens identity and harms emotional health. The evolution from patienthood to personhood is not necessarily a rejection of mental illness but rather an integration of its central experiences into a total self-image (Roe, 2001).

Self-identification is not a yes-no question; the decision is a bit grayer. On some issues, people may identify with mental illness entirely (e.g., the haunting impact of depression and/or dealing with the side effects of medication), while on other issues, they do not (e.g., anger with a restrictive mental health system). Moreover, ways in which people identify themselves with mental illness change over time. Mental illness may have different significance depending on whether psychiatric disabilities are still present, or whether a person has recently experienced the stigma of mental illness.

PRIDE AND IDENTITY

People who enjoy an identity have pride in it. Pride comes from a sense of accomplishment or rootedness. On one hand, people experience pride in achieving a standard recognized by their culture (e.g., a medal for the long-distance runner or a college degree for the person challenged by psychiatric disabilities) or set by themselves (e.g., a personal-best running time or meeting a course deadline when experiencing a recurrence of

WHAT'S THERE TO BE PROUD OF? This was the title of my chapter in *Coming Out Proud to Erase the Stigma of Mental Illness*, a collection of thirty-six stories of solidarity (Corrigan, Larson, & Michaels, 2015). Is *pride* a fair word here? After all, I dropped out of school (four times), got hospitalized, had side effects, and disappointed my family. Is this an accomplishment to wear on my sleeve with honor? There are other aspects of my identity that I proudly share. I am Pat Corrigan, a son, husband, father, psychologist, Irishman, Chicagoan . . . Depression and anxiety, what's to be proud of?

Somewhere along the way something changed. Mental illness became part of who I am. When and how I am not sure. But I noticed that over time I have included aspects of mental illness and recovery in pictures of myself. It has developed equal prominence in my story. Not everyone with mental health challenges does so; most people I treated in psychotherapy had symptoms that remitted, so they will go on with life untouched. Most of the research suggests they are right. However, there are other people who, as a result of their illness, corresponding treatments, and reactions of others, add mental illness and recovery to the self-statements that define who they are.

So I am a person with mental illness. Is this something to be proud of? Definitions of pride include two components: accomplishment and authenticity. Accomplishments are defined by external criteria as well as personal goals. I was proud when I came in first for my age group at the Morton Grove 5K race. I was also proud when I beat my personal-best time at a second 5K in Glenview. I have earned a doctorate in psychology, authored or edited more than a dozen books, and am distinguished faculty at my university. They are markers of accomplishment. However, victories inherent in overcoming my depression and anxiety trump those many fold. I remember being physically crushed and bent over when I got out of the hospital in 2005. I had two children in school and had to get back to work. A marathon seemed less daunting. But I did it. Getting back on my work feet surpassed all the challenges of grad school and faculty tenure.

Pride is also an issue of authenticity or embracing who you are. I am fourth-generation Irish American. My great grandfather came over to the Chicago area about one hundred years ago. I am fairly far removed from my Irish roots. But I am proud of being Irish American, especially every March 17 when Chicago dyes the river green. It is who I am, a part of my story that stands out for me.

I share an extra admission about authenticity. I am a trained operant and cognitive therapist with views about good therapy based on B. F. Skinner and Aaron Beck. I once ran a training center for Illinois, visiting state hospitals to set up token economies. Words like *authenticity* scared me, always seeming mushy and of no real value in helping people meet real-world goals. Authenticity scared me until I tried to make sense of who I am; why do I need to add experiences of illness and recovery to my stories of family and professional accomplishments? Authenticity for me is the full picture, nothing hidden. I admit that in weak moments authenticity still seems a little flaky as a therapy goal, something an existentialist (my god) might pursue rather than an evidence-based clinician. But as a human and friend and peer, authenticity—putting it out there who I am—has immense worth.

depression). Hence overcoming the challenges of mental illness may lead to identity pride, an experience not to be minimized. This view may have a downside, however, because it echoes the medical view of recovery, that pride is only achieved when symptoms abate and disabilities are resolved. An alternative perspective recognizes that a sense of agency and self-determination, in addition to the symptoms and disabilities of mental illness, fosters self-esteem and self-worth as part of an identity about which a person might be proud.

Pride also emerges from a sense of self. Ethnic pride is a clear example; the statement, "I am African American," does not suggest any accomplishment per se, but rather satisfaction with heritage, an additional answer to the question, Who am I? This phenomenon explains mental illness as an identity in which a person might be proud. This kind of identity promotes authenticity, a recognition of internal conceptualizations in the face of an imposing world. Authentic people are proud of their authenticity.

Group identification, defined as feelings of strong ties to a socially defined collection of people, has been shown to diminish the effects of stigma on people with mental illness. People with mental illness who identified more with the group of people labeled "mentally ill" were actually less likely to experience harm to self-esteem or self-efficacy as a result of internalized stigma (Watson, Corrigan, Larson, & Sells, 2007). Strong group identification was associated both with viewing stigma as potentially more harmful and with more perceived resources to cope with this threat. This means that identifying with the group of people with mental illness can both expose the individual to the risk of being discriminated against as a member of that group (the downside of disclosure) and offer sources of support to cope with discrimination (Rüsch et al., 2009a).

COMING OUT PROUD AS A PUBLIC HEALTH PROGRAM

How do public health advocates promote coming out? One program targeting this goal was developed for lesbians (Morrow, 1996). It was an ambitious self-help effort with ten sessions that addressed issues such as costs and benefits of living openly, homophobia communication skills, sexism assertiveness training, and workplace issues. Results of a nonexperimental study showed higher disclosure rates in the intervention than in the control group. Increased disclosure corresponded with lesbian identity development and enhanced personal empowerment. We developed *Honest, Open, Proud* (HOP) for public health advocates to help people with mental illness address disclosure and identity (Corrigan & Lundin, 2014). Program materials can be reviewed and downloaded for free at www .HOPprogram.org. HOP is a three-part program that addresses key issues related to disclosure: (1) costs and benefits of coming out, (2) strategic approaches to disclosure, and (3) crafting the personal story.

COSTS AND BENEFITS OF DISCLOSING

People with similar stories may still perceive differences in the costs and benefits of disclosure. Marie is thirty-two years old and has had more than a dozen years of struggling with schizophrenia. Despite this disability, things are working out well; she has not had a hospitalization in five years, she is working a good job, she is keeping a nice home, and she is living with a supportive husband. By many people's standards, she has beaten her mental illness. Still, Marie frequently attends mutual help groups where she provides support to peers who struggle with more acute problems related to their illness. She is also an outspoken advocate against stigma. She testifies at government hearings where she discloses as a person in recovery who is outraged by the disrespectful images of mental illness that are rampant in our society. *Marie is a person who identifies herself as "mentally ill."*

John Henry has similar history having struggled with schizophrenia since he was nineteen. Now, he is thirty-two, married, and working a great job in a law office. He has not been hospitalized in five years and almost no one at work or in his social circle knows about his illness. John Henry wants it that way. Not only does he choose not to let others know about his past, he does not view himself as a person with mental illness. "I'm a complex being with only a very small piece of me having to do with mental illness." *John Henry is a person who does not identify himself as "mentally ill."*

Openly disclosing one's experiences with mental illness is a complex decision that people need to make for themselves. In the example, two people with the same experiences view themselves and their mental illness differently. Marie thinks it is a significant part of her identity. John Henry denies mental illness as central to his core. Neither of their decisions is right or wrong. Instead, their choices represent their own analysis of the benefits and costs of disclosing. There are a variety of possible benefits and limitations to disclosure that might inform an individual's decision.

One advantage to disclosing is no longer having to worry about the secret getting out. It frees the person of the fear related to keeping secrets as well as of the resentment that stems from having to hide a part of oneself. Disclosing to other people helps the person to feel more open about day-to-day experiences. As a result, disclosure might yield approval and support from others. Most people are coping with some kind of personal trial or tribulation, even if it is not mental illness. They may be impressed by a person's ability to cope. Sometimes, people discover that when they admit to psychiatric problems, others respond with "me too." Disclosing may build friendships with those who have similar problems. These friends may then be available to help in the future. In fact, disclosing experiences with mental illness may be the first step to finding an entire support network of people with like problems.

Keeping a secret about mental illness fosters a feeling of shame. Telling one's story promotes a sense of power. A feeling of personal power is the opposite of being victimized by shame. Telling one's secret challenges many of the stigmatizing attitudes others have about mental illness. The person is living testimony against many of the said and unsaid myths about psychiatric disability.

Although there are benefits to disclosing, people need to also be aware of its costs. These costs are the force behind this entire book. One group of reasons why a person may choose not to disclose is the repercussions from others. Some people may disapprove of others telling their experiences. They fear mental illness or are offended by people who have been hospitalized. They may turn these emotions against you. Others may resent the person for asserting their right to tell. Some people might start talking about the person who discloses. Gossip is the bane of offices and neighborhoods. Telling people about experiences with depression, hospitals, or medications provides juicy material for the gossip line. As a result, some people are going to shun the individual who discloses at social gatherings when they hear their story. They may have ignorant views about people with mental illness being dangerous and want to protect themselves. Even worse, some people may exclude the individual from work or housing opportunities.

People who disclose may worry what others think because they told your secret. They wonder what people mean when they ask, "How are you?" or say they, "can't join you for lunch." Others may be concerned that people who find out will pity you. "It was bad enough to have to keep my history a secret. But I told a couple of guys from the local café and they were patronizing. 'Don't stress yourself, dear. Don't work too hard, buddy.' I would have rather had their scorn."

Disclosure is not a one-time decision. Depending on life circumstances, interests in disclosing change over time. People may decide today not to disclose but change their mind in a month. Disclosing experiences with mental illness is a journey, just like any important life decision. People constantly decide how much energy to spend on friends, family, work, and faith-based community. Sometimes, people are invested in work and ignore recreation. Other times, they focus on family and hobbies. The same variegations occur with disclosure.

People need to proceed with caution. Disclosure is solely the decision of individuals with serious mental illness about themselves. Although by nature I am progressive and liberal, believing guts and determination are essential to promoting social justice, I urge caution about disclosure. It is hard to stop the clanging bell. Once the person is out, it is hard to go back. Still, I know benefits of disclosing and believe it has value. There are relatively safe ways to do this.

STRATEGIC APPROACHES TO DISCLOSURE

Research summarized in the HOP program shows that disclosure is not a simple or solitary process but might be described by a hierarchy of five approaches (Herman, 1993).

1. Social avoidance: Ironically, the most basic way to handle disclosure may be to not tell anyone. This means avoiding situations where people may find out about one's mental illness. People who are victimized by stigma may choose not to socialize with, live near, or work alongside people without disabilities. Instead, they only associate with others who have mental illness. This may include people with mental illness living in a therapeutic community, working in a sheltered or supported work environment, or interacting with friends in a social club developed for mental illness. In this way, the person can avoid the "normal" population that may disapprove of their disabilities or actively work to keep them out.

In some ways, this approach is similar to old notions of *asylum*. A few people have such severe psychiatric disabilities that they need a safe and pleasant place to live and work, a place where they can escape the pressures and disapproval of society. What was known as the "moral view of psychiatric care" was originally envisioned by state hospitals: nice homes, rural settings, and supportive caretakers who help people with extreme disabilities to escape the stresses of society, as well as to escape those citizens in society who will stigmatize them. Unfortunately, few places ever achieved this goal, in part because most state and private facilities are dominated by patients with acute symptoms, some of whom might potentially be dangerous to themselves or others. They became custodial institutions, not open campuses where people can recover. The predominant concern for protection of patients from violence frequently overrides many of the "pleasant" aspects of hospital living.

This kind of asylum might be more appropriately accomplished in community-based programs. People with profound disabilities, who choose not to address their community's prejudice against mental illness, could live in pleasant compounds and work in sheltered settings away from the rest of their neighbors. People could learn to cope with their symptoms or achieve their interpersonal goals in a setting relatively free of disapproving neighbors or coworkers. Unfortunately, there are major negatives to social avoidance. People who choose to avoid the "normal" world miss out on benefits that it brings—free access to broader opportunities and citizens who support experience with mental illness. Social avoidance promotes stigma and discrimination. It endorses the idea that people with mental illness need to be locked away from the rest of the world. People who choose to avoid social situations may be putting off a challenge that they must eventually face. Social avoidance may be a useful strategy during times when symptoms are intense and the person needs a respite from demands of society. But, avoiding the normal world altogether will likely prevent most people from achieving the breadth of their life goals.

A more moderate approach to social avoidance might be to steer clear of certain groups of people—those who stigmatize—rather than steering clear of one's community as a whole. This requires being alert for people who are intolerant of individuals with mental illness. Avoid the bigot who looks at all people, especially minorities and disadvantaged groups, from a stereotyped, cruel, and disrespectful perspective. The "mentally ill" are derided by bigots who have contempt for everyone outside of their own narrow spectrum of acceptable people or races.

2. Secrecy: There is no need to avoid work or community situations in order to keep experiences with mental illness private. Many people choose to enter

these worlds, but to not share their experiences with others. Jose was a popular employee at a large food store for six years and never told coworkers he had been hospitalized for schizophrenia. Cynthia car-pooled her kids with neighbors for eighteen months and never let them know about her depression. Fariq went to mosque weekly and never let others know his history with bipolar disorder. It was not too hard for them to hide their psychiatric history.

Is this really possible? Sometimes, it seems like everyone can tell that a person is struggling with symptoms. The reality, however, is that experience with mental illness can be hidden. Keeping mental illness a secret is much easier than hiding one's gender, ethnic background, or physical disability. Experiences with psychosis and depression are private. Most people are unable to tell whether a coworker is hearing voices. They do not know a person's beliefs or emotions, unless told. Alternatively, many of the signs of mental illness are overlooked. Coworkers may think depression is temporary blues. Neighbors may think confusion is being sleepy-headed. There is a tendency in the human condition that protects privacy; most everyone is tuned into themselves, missing much of the psychological subtlety that surrounds them. Finally, many of the signs of mental illness are misunderstood. The public frequently labels eccentric or unusual conduct as wrong. People who are dressed poorly are homeless and "mentally ill." Individuals who punk their hair or pierce their ears are outlandish. People who dress within customary bounds will be overlooked.

3. Selective disclosure: When keeping experiences with mental illness secret, the person is not able to avail the support and resources of others. To rectify this problem, some people take a chance and disclose their mental illness to selected coworkers or neighbors. These people are taking a risk, however, because those who find out may shun them. With the risk comes opportunity. People who disclose may find people who are supportive. Moreover, the person will not have to worry about keeping a secret from those to whom you have disclosed. There are ways to "test" a person for safe disclosure with one method discussed next.

4. Indiscriminant disclosure: Selective disclosure means there is a group of people who know about one's mental illness experiences, *and* there is a group from whom the information is being kept secret. More than likely, the latter group is much larger than those with whom information has been

shared. This means there is still a large number of people whom the person does not want to find out about past experiences. Moreover, there is still a secret that could represent a source of shame. People who choose indiscriminant disclosure abandon this secrecy. They choose to disregard any of the potential negative consequences of people finding out about their mental illness. The decision to no longer conceal is not the same as telling everyone the story. Not keeping a secret means that the person is no longer trying to hide it. The person is relieved of the burden posed by the secret. Indiscriminant disclosure requires a hardy personality. Many other people are going to find out and react negatively to your mental illness. The person disclosing experiences needs to cope with the disapproval that results from bigoted reactions.

5. Broadcast your experience: Indiscriminant disclosure means no longer trying to hide one's mental illness. Still, people are not likely to go out of their way to inform others about it. Broadcasting means educating people about mental illness. It is like coming out of the closet in the gay community; the goal is to actively let people know about mental illness through a first-person voice. This kind of disclosure is much more than dropping guard and throwing away secrecy. The goal is to seek out many people with whom to share your past history and current experiences with mental illness.

Broadcasting has the same benefits as indiscriminant disclosure. People no longer worry about keeping a secret. They also find others who may provide understanding, support, and assistance because of the message. People who choose to broadcast their experience seem to derive an additional benefit. It fosters a sense of power over the experience of mental illness and stigma. No longer must they cower because of feelings of inferiority. Shouting this out relieves people of community oppression. In fact, many people who choose to broadcast their experience wish to surpass the limited goal of talking about their mental illness. They also express their dissatisfaction with the way they have been treated because they have a mental illness. This discontent is also aimed at society: anger at being viewed differently, losing opportunities, and having to keep secrets.

Broadcasting experiences may yield hostile responses, just like indiscriminate disclosure. Members of the "normal" majority who hear someone's story about mental illness frequently battle the message and the messenger. Like the person choosing indiscriminate disclosure, broadcasters get hostile reactions to their messages. "Why do I have to live next to a crazy guy like you? You're dangerous to my family. I'll be keeping an eye on you." Civil rights leaders have experienced similar reactions. Challenging messages from racial groups about economic equality and political injustice upset the status quo. People in power do not want to hear this. In a similar manner, talking about mental illness and displeasure with society's reactions is disquieting. Citizens may rebel against the messenger with angry denials.

TESTING SOMEONE FOR DISCLOSURE

People seeking to share their experiences might test someone to determine if they are a good person for disclosure. The HOP program provides one way to do this. They might do this by first writing down an example from recent news stories, magazine articles, TV shows, or movies related to mental illness, and then share it with a friend. The goal is to share something benign: "Did you see the movie *Silver Linings Playbook* with Bradley Cooper and Jennifer Lawrence?" This provides a safe opportunity to find out what the person thinks about mental illness. Benign is important. A discussion about a mass shooting like the tragedy at Sandy Hook Elementary School where twenty children and six adults were shot dead by Adam Lanza will only evoke stigma. Ask the person, "what did you think?" If they respond, "I am sick and tired of these kinds of crybaby shows where they make mental illness look noble," one learns this person is likely a bad candidate for disclosure. Alternatively, people who respond, "I thought Bradley Cooper and Jennifer Lawrence portrayed mental illness honestly," might be good people to disclose to. Follow-up with a question like, "Do you know anyone with bipolar disorder like Bradley Cooper acted out?"

CRAFTING ONE'S STORY

A decision to disclose does not mean disclose everything. Disclosure does not mean giving up all of one's privacy. Just as people must decide to whom they disclose, so they decide what will be shared. Through the HOP program, people determine which experiences in the past to discuss and what current experiences they want to keep private. The purpose of disclosing the past is to give people some knowledge of problems with mental illness. The goal is not confession. Everyone has skeletons in their closet; the person does not have to air their skeletons in order to get others to understand that they have recovered from a serious mental illness. Specific issues they may wish to share include: diagnosis, symptoms, history of hospitalizations, and medications.

> I have a serious mental illness called schizophrenia. As a result, I have heard voices, had some strange beliefs, and been agitated. I was hospitalized four times in two years because of this. My psychiatrist and I have tried several different medications. Right now, my symptoms are managed well by a drug called Zyprexa.

Notice the words "may wish to share." All people decide for themselves.

The purpose of sharing current experiences is twofold. First, the individual may want to impress upon others that the serious mental illness of long ago has much less impact on now; "I can control small problems that occur in my life." Although mental illness may not go away entirely, the person is still able to work, raise a family, and be a responsible member of society. The second goal is to alert others that the individual may have troubles in the future and need some assistance.

ADAPTING HOP FOR DIFFERENT COMMUNITIES

The process of disclosure is socially constructed; it is implemented and received differently depending on the community in which it occurs. Hence, programs such as *Honest, Open, Proud* need to be adapted for different communities. One way community may be defined is by condition. People with serious mental illness come together as a community to erase stigma separate from people with substance use disorders. Community may be defined by age; young people likely view stigma and its impact differently than those in their senior years. Stigma varies by ethnicity and religion such that, for example, anti-stigma efforts for Muslims are likely to differ than those for Christians.

Adapting HOP or any anti-stigma program so it specifically represents the interests of individual groups is done using community-based participatory research (CBPR). The importance of CBPR was highlighted at the end of chapter 2 when describing effective ways to evaluate anti-stigma programs. CBPR is led by a team of partners: people with lived experience, their allies, and researchers. The first two groups are essential for developing a program that represents the perceived interest of the group. Hence, programs meant to erase the stigma of addiction should be led by people with substance use disorders. This could include people with current disorders and those in recovery. CBPR teams also include allies. This likely includes not only family and friends but also service providers. Researchers bring the technical skills necessary to complete anti-stigma program development in a reliable and valid manner. As a result, the CBPR team develops anti-stigma programs that represent lived perceptions of stigma's harm and effective ways to erase it. Ownership is an essential byproduct. Instead of a program that comes from an ivory tower of academics with limited knowledge of harm, the program comes from those with lived experience who then assume responsibility for disseminating the intervention outside the team.

Consider the complexity of this task. Our research group has recently come together to develop HOP for South Asians. India is one country in South Asia and is dominated by Hindus (about 80 percent of the population), but also has large numbers of Muslims (14.2 percent), Christians (2.3 percent), and Sikhs (1.7 percent) (Census of India, 2011). These religious groups are spread over 2000 ethnic groups, speaking languages from four major families: Indo-European, Dravidian, Austroasiatic, and Sino-Tibetan (Central Intelligence Agency, 2017). There are conceivably thousands of CBPR teams for a community harmed by differing behavioral health stigma. CBPR to adapt HOP will occur when those groups identify stigma as a problem for them and decide to craft a program specific to their needs.

Disclosure and age is also an important focus for program development. Young people share much of their story on social media. This might include online video chat, in which information is exchanged via the Internet. Popular examples include Skype or FaceTime. There are benefits to using online video chat, such as the ability to express emotion and to observe

In 2015, we conducted Honest, Open, Proud for inmates in the Cook County Jail (CCJ). The jail houses people awaiting trial or serving short sentences from Chicago and surrounding suburbs. CCJ is one of the largest providers of mental health services in the United States because the criminal justice system nets large numbers of people with mental illness who are arrested or found guilty for relatively minor crimes. Typically, inmates are African American males. HOP seemed to be a natural intervention for CCJ inmates with serious mental illness.

In the first meeting, we engaged inmates in HOP exercises about understanding pros and cons of disclosing past mental health experiences. They were able to make a typical list, but discussion soon got derailed to tangential stigma.

- "Sure, the stigma of mental illness is bad, but what about the fact that I also abuse drugs? My family doesn't like that."
- "And I got HIV-AIDS. Everyone thinks I'm a gay pervert that is going to infect them with a disease."
- "Let's not forget that everyone in this room is an inmate; we are tagged as criminal, with a warning sign that leads to all sorts of discrimination when we get out."
- "It's all made worse because I didn't get very far in school. I'm not even a high school graduate. Everyone thinks I'm stupid."

This experience highlighted how intersectionality challenges HOP. With which of these conditions does the group begin? Self-determination seems to be a natural way to answer this question. Let the group decide. But, for example, if the group decides to unpack the stigma of HIV-AIDS and the risk of disclosure, what happens to group members who are not HIV positive?

reactions from others. The person will also be speaking in real time, so it might be wise to plan one's message. The second kind of social media is private messages such as text messages, e-mails, and private Facebook messages. This venue makes disclosure less stressful: the person does not have to "look the person in the eye" and disclose, but instead tells the person privately over a carefully thought-out message. Sending the message privately does not mean it will stay private. Unlike online video chat, written messages can be shared with others whether they want them to be or not.

The final category of social media that can be used for disclosure is media such as Twitter, Instagram, blog posts, and public Facebook statuses where public messages might be posted. This type of disclosure should only be used if the person is trying to broadcast experience to anyone and is not fazed by who knows about their mental illness. Benefits of this include finally being "out" to everyone, freeing one's self from keeping secrets from others, and having an opportunity to educate the public about one's mental illness. This kind of post might also get negative comments from people disapproving of the message. Note that there is no prescription here on whether and how youth might post their experiences with mental illness on social media. Instead, programs like HOP need to provide a venue among peers where pros and cons of different e-disclosures can be considered. Individuals can then decide how to proceed on their pages given this information.

8

LESSONS LEARNED FOR
FUTURE ADVOCACY

T
HE EXISTING BODY of research and experience on stigma and stigma
change has led to several lessons that should guide future work in
this area. These are lessons to help people avoid the stigma effect and
make real changes in the injustices that face people with mental illness.
First, there should be no doubt that stigma is a major problem for people
with mental illness and related behavioral health disorders. Stigma can
be more harmful to people than the illness itself. It is not secondary to
the more primary challenges of symptoms and should not be relegated to the
back seat with public health focusing solely on symptom and disability management. It will not go away when mental illness is cured. Stigma is a
complex phenomenon with anti-stigma efforts needing to understand and
differentiate between the egregious effects of public and self-stigma, label
avoidance, structural stigma, and stigma by association. Ending stigma is
by no means sufficient; social justice is achieved only when affirming attitudes such as recovery and self-determination, and affirming behaviors such
as reasonable accommodations and community opportunities, become the
dominant descriptors for serious mental illness.

The good news is that many progressive people understand stigma's
harmful effects and organize together in order to stop it. At times, however, this leads to unintended mistakes. Advocates avoid mistakes by first
understanding the differing reasons for challenging stigma defined by services, rights, and self-worth agenda. Each agenda has value but can work

at cross-purposes with the others. For example, anti-stigma programs addressing a services agenda might promote messages like "depression is a medical disorder than can be treated effectively by medication and psychotherapy" and may unintentionally perpetuate the idea that individuals who are depressed are "sick." Sick people are different from the "normal" majority; this perceived difference exacerbates discrimination leading to loss of rights in work, education, and independent-living situations.

With eagerness and zeal, progressives charge into the stigma arena at times with interventions that not only fail to have benefit but may actually worsen outcomes. Two examples are especially notable: (1) Just change the words! The call for different language is an easy but ineffective way to meaningfully challenge stigma. Language-change programs are lost opportunities distracting people from more effective approaches to stigma change. (2) Educate away stigma with new information! At least for adults, new information about behavioral health challenges does not change stigma. Improving mental health literacy may have some value for individuals who do not understand distressing experiences as treatable mental health conditions. But it does not diminish prejudice that the "normal" majority has against those with mental health challenges.

Person-to-person interaction is the way to decrease the stigma of mental illness. Hostile attitudes between ethnic groups diminish when people from those groups interact as peers. Racist attitudes against African Americans have diminished to the extent that blacks and whites exchange perceptions of their world as equals. The stigma of many groups is hidden, however. Members of the lesbian, gay, bisexual, transgender, questioning (LGBTQ) community, for example, may not be stigmatized unless they disclose or are somehow outed. Hence, people who have come out with their sexual orientation, and interacted with the straight community as peers, have been the heroes of gay rights efforts. Note how stigma has been dampened here. Younger generations have been able to throw off homophobic ideas about LGBTQ community members, *not* because they learned in high school health class that sexual orientation is genetic and not chosen. They escaped the tyranny of homophobia because courageous gays and lesbians came out forty to fifty years ago. While growing up, our youth were able to interact with a gay uncle, lesbian family friend, bisexual teacher, or gay political figure.

The stigma of mental illness will equally lessen when men and women with behavioral health challenges come out. Stigma will be replaced by affirming attitudes when the "normal" majority interacts with people with mental illness as equals. In this way, the "normal" majority learns that people with mental illness have a set of diverse hopes and aspirations that are achievable. This means that people with mental illness need to disclose their mental illness. The atomic bomb to erase stigma is to come out. Coming out, however, has its risks. I would never encourage anyone to ignore these risks and blithely share experiences with mental health challenges. Coming out, however, can help individuals overcome the shame of mental illness. The process is easier when the person considers costs, benefits, and strategies with peers who are on a similar journey.

Anti-stigma programs need to be led by people with lived experience, not by their allies. This may suggest a change in direction for some programs. Family members and service providers, being key advocates for those with serious mental illness, have stepped up in the past to assert community rights for those in their care. However, stigma efforts now need to be led by those who are harmed by the prejudice and discrimination. I am a straight male who unequivocally endorses LGBTQ rights. However, programs that push those rights need to be led by members of the LGBTQ community. Straights are their allies. Similarly, programs addressing the harm caused by mental illness stigma must be led by those with lived experience.

There is not a litmus test that defines the bar at which people qualify as sufficiently "mentally" ill to have lived experience, to be an anti-stigma advocate. People who identify with mental illness—who know the shame and discrimination—and who are motivated to tear down the stigma, are people with lived experience. Typically, these are individuals who have experienced serious psychiatric symptoms over prolonged time that have been disabling. They may be people who have experienced invasive therapies or social opprobrium from their network, all of which led to a growing realization of the harmful effects of stigma. However, some people come to identify with the stigma after a relatively benign course of mental illness. Perhaps a person with an adjustment disorder that occurs after the death of a loved one experiences an unexpected shame that results from the "mental illness label." This may be sufficient for them to identify with the group of people with lived experience and join anti-stigma efforts.

Repeatedly throughout the book I have said that stigma is a social construction. As such, stigma and stigma change are likely to be experienced differently by different social groups: ethnicity, religion, gender, sexual orientation, and age, to name a few. Hence, one program will not fit all. A disclosure program will no doubt vary between Americans and South Asians. This may mean advocates need to take the time to make sure an anti-stigma effort addresses the preferences of the group in which it is immersed. Community-based participatory research (CBPR) may be needed. This is not a trivial consideration. There are already developed, empirically validated approaches for erasing the stigma of some behavioral health disorders. Advocates have an urgency to their work, wanting to adopt these approaches so injustices can be removed now. Perhaps a quick tweak will allow them to do this. Alternatively, a more deliberate CBPR effort might be needed. Only people from the group of interest can decide.

Earlier, I described myself as a 1960s voyeur; I was too young to join college students in the streets marching against racism and the Vietnam War, but I took in the drama on the nightly news. I was enthralled by progressives who saw the injustice of the moment and came together to change the social order. They did this raucously and with optimism. I was a 1960s progressive before I became a mental health advocate, and those memories drive my effort to make changes to communities that can be hostile to people with mental health challenges. I encourage the reader to draw on their personal source of optimism to join in the anti-stigma effort. I encourage them to be critical in their efforts, to make sure their optimism is not blind but is informed by empowering approaches that make real change in the stigmatizing status quo.

REFERENCES

Aboud, F. E. (1988). *Children and prejudice.* New York: B. Blackwell.

Aboud, F. E. (2003). The formation of in-group favoritism and out-group prejudice in young children: Are they distinct attitudes? *Developmental Psychology, 39*(1), 48–60.

Aboud, F. E., & Doyle, A. B. (1996). Parental and peer influences on children's racial attitudes. *International Journal of Intercultural Relations, 20*(3–4), 371–383.

Aboud, F. E., & Fenwick, V. (1999). Exploring and evaluating school-based interventions to reduce prejudice. *Journal of Social Issues, 55*(4), 767–785.

Aboud, F. E., & Levy, S. R. (2000). Interventions to reduce prejudice and discrimination in children and adolescents. In S. Oskamp (Ed.), *Reducing prejudice and discrimination* (pp. 269–293). Mahwah, NJ: Lawrence Erlbaum Associates, Inc.

Abrams, D., & Hogg, M. A. (1988). Comments on the motivational status of self-esteem in social identity and intergroup discrimination. *European Journal of Social Psychology, 18*(4), 317–334.

Allport, G. W. (1954). *The nature of prejudice.* Reading, MA: Addison-Wesley.

Allport, G. W. (1979). *The nature of prejudice.* Reading, MA: Addison-Wesley.

American Psychiatric Association. (2013). *Diagnostic and statistical manual of mental disorders* (5th ed.). Arlington, VA: American Psychiatric Publishing.

Americans with Disabilities Act of 1990, Pub. L. No. 101–336, 104 Stat. 328 (1990).

Augoustinos, M., & Rosewarne, D. L. (2001). Stereotype knowledge and prejudice in children. *British Journal of Developmental Psychology, 19*(1), 143–156.

Beals, K. P., Peplau, L. A., & Gable, S. L. (2009). Stigma management and well-being: The role of perceived social support, emotional processing, and suppression. *Personality and Social Psychology Bulletin, 35*(7), 867–879.

Beers, C. (1909). *The after care of the insane.* New Haven, CT: Bradley & Scoville.

Bell, J., Colangelo, A., & Pillen, M. (2005). *Final report of the evaluation of the elimination of barriers initiative.* Arlington, VA: James Bell Associates.

Bettelheim, B., & Janowitz, M. (1964). *Social change and prejudice.* Oxford, UK: Free Press Glencoe.

Biernat, M., & Dovidio, J. F. (2000). Stigma and stereotypes. In T. F. Heatherton (Ed.), *The social psychology of stigma* (pp. 88–125). New York: Guilford Press.

Bonovitz, J. C., & Bonovitz, J. S. (1981). Diversion of the mentally ill into the criminal justice system: The police intervention perspective. *American Journal of Psychiatry, 138*(7), 973–976.

Branscombe, N. R., Schmitt M. T., & Harvey R. D. (1999). Perceiving pervasive discrimination among African Americans: Implications for group identification and well-being. *Journal of Personality and Social Psychology, 77*(1), 135–149.

Breggin, P., & Breggin, G. R. (1994). *Talking back to Prozac: What doctors won't tell you about today's most controversial drug.* New York: St. Martin's Paperbacks.

Brown, C. S., Markowitz, J. S., Moore, T. R., & Parker, N. G. (1999). Atypical antipsychotics: Part II adverse effects, drug interactions, and costs. *Annals of Pharmacotherapy, 33*(2), 210–217.

Buchanan, R. W., Kreyenbuhl, J., Kelly, D. L., Noel, J. M., Boggs, D. L., Fischer, B. A., . . . Keller, W. (2010). The 2009 schizophrenia PORT psychopharmacological treatment recommendations and summary statements. *Schizophrenia Bulletin, 36*(1), 71–93.

Calabrese, J. D., & Corrigan, P. W. (2005). Beyond dementia praecox: Findings from long-term follow-up studies of schizophrenia. In R. O. Ralph, P. W. Corrigan (Eds.), *Recovery in mental illness: Broadening our understanding of wellness* (pp. 63–84). Washington, DC: American Psychological Association. doi: 10.1037/10848-003

Census of India. (2011). *C-1 population by religious community* [Data file]. Retrieved from http://www.censusindia.gov.in/2011census/C-01.html

Centers for Disease Control and Prevention. (2016). National Vital Statistics System, Mortality. CDC WONDER. Atlanta, GA: US Department of Health and Human Services. https://wonder.cdc.gov/wonder/help/ucd.html#

Centers for Disease Control and Prevention. (2017). Measles cases and outbreaks. *MMWR. Morbidity and Mortality Weekly Reports.* Retrieved from https://www.cdc.gov/measles/cases-outbreaks.html

Centers for Disease Control and Prevention: The Community Guide. (2010). *Mental health and mental illness: Collaborative care for the management of depressive disorders.* Retrieved from https://www.thecommunityguide.org/findings/mental-health-and-mental-illness-collaborative-care-management-depressive-disorders

Central Intelligence Agency. (2017). *India demographics profile.* Retrieved from https://www.cia.gov/library/publications/the-world-factbook/

Chae, J., Lee, C. J., & Jensen, J. D. (2016). Correlates of cancer information overload: Focusing on individual ability and motivation. *Health Communication, 31*(5), 626–634.

Chamberlin, J. (1978). *On our own: Patient-controlled alternatives to the mental health system.* New York: Haworth Press.

Chinman, M., Salzer, M., & O'Brien-Mazza, D. (2012). National survey on implementation of peer specialists in the VA: Implications for training and facilitation. *Psychiatric Rehabilitation Journal, 35,* 470–473.

Christopher Reeve, thrown from horse, is suffering paralysis. (1995, June 1). *New York Times.* Retrieved from http://www.nytimes.com/1995/06/01/us/christopher-reeve-thrown-from-horse-is-suffering-paralysis.html

Corrigan, P. W. (2016). *The principles and practice of psychiatric rehabilitation: An empirical approach* (2nd ed.). New York: Guilford Press.

Corrigan, P. W., Angell, B., Davidson, L., Marcus, S. C., Salzer, M. S., Kottsieper, P., . . . Stanhope, V. (2012). From adherence to self-determination: Evolution of a treatment paradigm for people with serious mental illnesses. *Psychiatric Services*, *63*(2), 169–173. doi:10.1176/ appi.ps.201100065

Corrigan, P. W., & Fong, M. W. (2014). Competing perspectives on erasing the stigma of illness: What says the dodo bird? *Social Science & Medicine*, *103*, 110–117.

Corrigan, P. W., Kosyluk, K. A., Fokuo, J. K., & Park, J. H. (2014). How does direct to consumer advertising affect the stigma of mental illness? *Community Mental Health Journal*, *50*(7), 792–799.

Corrigan, P. W., Larson, J. E., & Michaels, P. J. (2015). *Coming out proud to erase the stigma of mental illness: Stories and essays of solidarity*. Collierville, TN: Instant Publisher.

Corrigan, P. W., & Lundin, R. (2014). *Coming out proud to eliminate the stigma of mental illness manual*. Retrieved from http://www.comingoutproudprogram.org/index.php/manual-and -resources

Corrigan, P. W., Michaels, P. J., & Morris, S. (2015). Do the effects of antistigma programs persist over time? Findings from a meta-analysis. *Psychiatric Services*, *66*(5), 543–546.

Corrigan, P. W., Morris, S., Larson, J., Rafacz, J., Wassell, A., Michaels, P., . . . Rusch, N. (2010). Self-stigma and coming out about one's mental illness. *Journal of Community Psychology*, *38*, 259–275.

Corrigan, P. W., Morris, S. B., Michaels, P. J., Rafacz, J. D., & Rusch, N. (2012). Challenging the public stigma of mental illness: A meta-analysis of outcome studies. *Psychiatric Services*, *63*, 963–973.

Corrigan, P. W., River, L. P., Lundin, R. K., Wasowski, K. U., Campion, J., Mathisen, J., . . . Kubiak, M. A. (2000). Stigmatizing attributions about mental illness. *Journal of Community Psychology*, *28*(1), 91–102.

Corrigan, P. W., & Shapiro, J. R. (2010). Measuring the impact of programs that challenge the public stigma of mental illness. *Clinical Psychology Review*, *30*(8), 907–922.

Crenshaw, K. W., Gotanda, N., Peller, G., & Thomas, K. (Eds.). (1995). *Critical race theory: Key writings that formed the movement*. New York: New Press.

Davidson, L. (2003). *Living outside mental illness: Qualitative studies of recovery in schizophrenia*. New York: New York University Press.

Davidson, L., Bellamy, C., Guy, K., & Miller, R. (2012). Peer support among persons with severe mental illnesses: A review of evidence and experience. *World Psychiatry*, *11*(2), 123–128.

Deegan, P. E. (1990). Spirit breaking: When the helping professions hurt. *Humanistic Psychologist*, *18*, 301–313.

DeJong, W., Wolf, R., & Austin, S. (2001). U.S. federally funded television public service announcements (PSAs) to prevent HIV/AIDS: A content analysis. *Journal of Health Communication*, *6*(3), 249–263.

Derman-Sparks, L., & Phillips, C. B. (1997). *Teaching/learning anti-racism: A developmental approach*. New York: Teachers College Press.

Dion, K. L. (2002). The social psychology of perceived prejudice and discrimination. *Canadian Psychology/Psychologie Canadienne*, *43*(1), 1.

Draine, J., Salzer, M. S., Culhane, D. P., & Hadley, T. R. (2002). Role of social disadvantage in crime, joblessness, and homelessness among persons with serious mental illness. *Psychiatric Services*, *53*(5), 565–573. doi:10.1176/appi.ps.53.5.565

Drake, R. E., Goldman, H. E., Leff, H. S., Lehman, A. F., Dixon, L., Mueser, K. T., & Torrey, W. C. (2001). Implementing evidence-based practices in routine mental health service settings. *Psychiatric Services, 52*(2), 179–182. doi:10.1176/appi.ps.52.2.179

Druss, B. G., Bradford, D. W., Rosenheck, R. A., Radford, M. J., & Krumholz, H. M. (2000). Mental disorders and use of cardiovascular procedures after myocardial infarction. *Journal of the American Medical Association, 283*(4), 506–511.

Escher, S., & Romme, M. (2012). The hearing voices movement. In *Hallucinations* (pp. 385–393). New York: Springer.

Evans, A., & Bosworth, K. (1998). Building effective drug education programs. *Phi Delta Kappa International, 19*, 1–10.

Fein, S., & Spencer, S. J. (1997). Prejudice as self-image maintenance: Affirming the self through derogating others. *Journal of Personality and Social Psychology, 73*(1), 31.

Flavell, J. H. (1999). Cognitive development: Children's knowledge about the mind. *Annual Review of Psychology, 50*(1), 21–45.

Fominaya, A. W., Corrigan, P. W., & Rüsch, N. (2016). The effects of pity on self- and other-perceptions of mental illness. *Psychiatry Research, 241*, 159–164.

Garstka, T. A., Schmitt, M. T., Branscombe, N. R., & Hummert, M. L. (2004). How young and older adults differ in their responses to perceived age discrimination. *Psychology and Aging, 19*(2), 326–335.

Goffman, E. (1963). *Stigma: Notes on the management of spoiled identity*. New York: Simon and Schuster.

Goldman, L., & Glantz, S. (1998). Evaluation of antismoking advertising campaigns. *Journal of the American Medical Association, 279*(10), 772–777.

Goldstrom, I., Campbell, J., Rogers, J., Lambert, D., Blacklow, B., Henderson, M., & Manderscheid, R. (2006). National estimates for mental health mutual support groups, self-help organizations, and consumer-operated services. *Administration and Policy in Mental Health., 33*(1), 92–103.

Gottschaldt, M. (1997). *Alcohol and pharmaceuticals. Ways to leave addiction. What is forming our Life: Addiction as an emotional problem* [in German]. Stuttgart: Georg Thieme Verlag.

Gove, W. R. (1975). *The labelling of deviance: Evaluating a perspective*. New York: John Wiley & Sons.

Grohmann, R., Engel, R. R., Geissler, K. H., & Rüther, E. (2004). Psychotropic drug use in psychiatric inpatients: Recent trends and changes over time-data from the AMSP study. *Pharmacopsychiatry, 37*(S1), 27–38.

Guttman, N., & Salmon, C. T. (2004). Guilt, fear, stigma and knowledge gaps: Ethical issues in public health communication interventions. *Bioethics, 18*(6), 531–552.

Hadlaczky, G., Hokby, S., Mkrtchian, A., Carli, V., & Wasserman, D. (2014). Mental Health First Aid is an effective public health intervention for improving knowledge, attitudes, and behavior. A meta-analysis. *International Review of Psychiatry, 26*(4), 467–475.

Halpin, S. A., & Allen, M. W. (2004). Changes in psychosocial well-being during stages of gay identity development. *Journal of Homosexuality, 47*(2), 109–126.

Harding, C. M., Brooks, G. W., Ashikaga, T., Strauss, J. S., & Breier, A. (1987a). The Vermont longitudinal study of persons with severe mental illness: I. Methodology, study sample, and overall status 32 years later. *American Journal of Psychiatry, 144*(6), 718–726.

Harding, C. M., Brooks, G. W., Ashikaga, T., Strauss, J. S., & Breier, A. (1987b). The Vermont longitudinal study of persons with severe mental illness: II. Long-term outcome of subjects who retrospectively met DSM-III criteria for schizophrenia. *American Journal of Psychiatry, 144*(6), 727–735.

Harrison, G., Hopper, K. I. M., Craig, T., Laska, E., Siegel, C., Wanderling, J., . . . Holmberg, S. K. (2001). Recovery from psychotic illness: A 15- and 25-year international follow-up study. *British Journal of Psychiatry, 178*(6), 506–517.

Hayes, S. C., Strosahl, K. D., & Wilson, K. G. (1999). *Acceptance and commitment therapy: An experiential approach to behavior change.* New York: Guilford Press.

Herek, G. M. (2007). Confronting sexual stigma and prejudice: Theory and practice. *Journal of Social Issues, 63*(4), 905–925.

Herman, N. J. (1993). Return to sender: Reintegrative stigma-management strategies of ex-psychiatric patients. *Journal of Contemporary Ethnography, 22*(3), 295–330.

Highet, N. J., Luscombe, G. M., Davenport, T. A., Burns, J. M., & Hickie, I. B. (2006). Positive relationships between public awareness activity and recognition of the impacts of depression in Australia. *Australian and New Zealand Journal of Psychiatry, 40*(1), 55–58.

Howarth, C. (2006). Race as stigma: Positioning the stigmatized as agents, not objects. *Journal of Community & Applied Social Psychology, 16*(6), 442–451.

Institute of Medicine. (2007). *Informing the future: Critical issues in health* (4th ed.). Washington, DC: National Academies Press.

Jensen, A. (1969). How much can we boost IQ and scholastic achievement? *Harvard Educational Review, 39*(1), 1–123.

Johnson, F. H. (1978). *The anatomy of hallucinations.* Oxford, UK: Nelson-Hall.

Jorm, A. F. (2012). Mental health literacy: Empowering the community to take action for better mental health. *American Psychologist, 67*(3), 231.

Jorm, A. F., Christensen, H., & Griffiths, K. M. (2005). The impact of beyondblue: the national depression initiative on the Australian public's recognition of depression and beliefs about treatments. *Australian and New Zealand Journal of Psychiatry, 39*(4), 248–254.

Jorm, A. F., & Kitchener, B. A. (2011). Noting a landmark achievement: Mental health first aid training reaches 1% of Australian adults. *Australian and New Zealand Journal of Psychiatry, 45*(10), 808–813.

Jost, J. T., Burgess, D., & Mosso, C. (1999). *Crises of legitimization among self, group, and system: A theoretical integration.* Graduate School of Business, Stanford University.

Lieberman, J. A., & Stroup, T. S. (2011). The NIMH-CATIE Schizophrenia Study: What did we learn? *American Journal of Psychiatry, 168*(8), 770–775.

Kabat-Zinn, J. (2013). Mindfulness-based interventions in medicine and psychiatry: What does it mean to be 'mindfulness-based'? In A. Fraser, A. Fraser (Eds.), *The healing power of meditation: Leading experts on Buddhism, psychology, and medicine explore the health benefits of contemplative practice* (pp. 93–119). Boston, MA: Shambhala Publications.

Kahneman, D. (1973). *Attention and effort* (p. 246). Englewood Cliffs, NJ: Prentice-Hall.

Katz, P. A., Sohn, M., & Zalk, S. R. (1975). Perceptual concomitants of racial attitudes in urban grade-school children. *Developmental Psychology, 11*(2), 135–144.

Katz, P. A., & Zalk, S. R. (1978). Modification of children's racial attitudes. *Developmental Psychology, 14*(5), 447.

Kenneson, A., Funderburk, J. S., & Maisto, S. A. (2013). Substance use disorders increase the odds of subsequent mood disorders. *Drug & Alcohol Dependence*, *133*(2), 338–343. doi:10.1016/j.drugalcdep.2013.06.011

Kessler, R. C., Berglund, P. A., Bruce, M. L., Koch, J. R., Laska, E. M., Leaf, P. J., . . . Wang, P. S. (2001). The prevalence and correlates of untreated serious mental illness. *Health Services Research*, *36*(6), 987–1007.

Kessler, R. C., & Merikangas, K. R. (2004). The National Comorbidity Survey Replication (NCS-R): Background and aims. *International Journal of Methods in Psychiatric Research*, *13*(2), 60–68. doi:10.1002/mpr.166

Kessler, R. C., Nelson, C. B., McGonagle, K. A., Edlund, M. J., Frank, R. G., & Leaf, P. J. (1996). The epidemiology of co-occurring addictive and mental disorders: Implications for prevention and service utilization. *American Journal of Orthopsychiatry*, *66*(1), 17–31. doi:10.1037/h0080151

King Jr., M. L. (14 March 1968). Up north: Martin Luther King, Jr., in Grosse Pointe. Grosse Pointe, Michigan. Available at www.gphistorical.org/mlk/mlkspeech/index.htm

Kotler, P., Roberto, N., & Lee, N. (2002). *Social marketing: Improving the quality of life*. Thousand Oaks, CA: SAGE Publications.

Kraepelin, E. (1896). *Psychiatrie. 5te Aufl*. Oxford, UK: J. A. Barth.

Kuhn, T. S. (1962). *The structure of scientific revolutions*. Chicago: University of Chicago Press.

Lally, S. J. (1989). "Does being in here mean there is something wrong with me?" *Schizophrenia Bulletin*, *15*(2), 253–265.

Larimer, M. E., Palmer, R. S., & Marlatt, G. A. (1999). Relapse prevention: An overview of Marlatt's cognitive-behavioral model. *Alcohol Research and Health*, *23*(2), 151–160.

Lefley, H. (2003). Advocacy, self-help, and consumer-operated services. In A. Tasman, J. Kay, & J. Lieberman (Eds.), *Psychiatry* (2nd ed., pp. 2274–2288). West Sussex, UK: John Wiley and Sons.

Liberman, R. P. (2008). Principles and practice of psychiatric rehabilitation: An empirical approach. *American Journal of Psychiatry*, *165*(7), 924–925.

Lieberman, J. A., & Stroup, T. S. (2011). The NIMH-CATIE Schizophrenia Study: What did we learn? *American Journal of Psychiatry*, *168*(8), 770–775.

Lienemann, B. A., Siegel, J. T., & Crano, W. D. (2013). Persuading people with depression to seek help: Respect the boomerang. *Health Communication*, *28*(7), 718–728.

Link, B. G. (1987). Understanding labeling effects in the area of mental disorders: An assessment of the effects of expectations of rejection. *American Sociological Review*, *52*(1), 96–112.

Link, B. G., Andrews, H., & Cullen, F. T. (1992). The violent and illegal behavior of mental patients reconsidered. *American Sociological Review*, 275–292.

Link, B. G., Mirotznik, J., & Cullen, F. T. (1991). The effectiveness of stigma coping orientations: Can negative consequences of mental illness labeling be avoided? *Journal of Health and Social Behavior*, *32*(3) 302–320.

Loury, G. C. (2005). Racial stigma and its consequences. *Focus*, *24*(1), 1–6.

Luborsky, L., Singer, B., & Luborsky, L. (1975). Comparative studies of psychotherapies: Is it true that everyone has won and all must have prizes? *Archives of General Psychiatry*, *32*(8), 995–1008.

Lucksted, A., Drapalski, A., Calmes, C., Forbes, C., DeForge, B., & Boyd, J. (2011). Ending self-stigma: Pilot evaluation of a new intervention to reduce internalized stigma among people with mental illnesses. *Psychiatric Rehabilitation Journal*, *35*(1), 51.

Lysaker, P. H., Davis, L. W., Warman, D. M., Strasburger, A., & Beattie, N. (2007). Stigma, social function and symptoms in schizophrenia and schizoaffective disorder: Associations across 6 months. *Psychiatry research*, *149*(1), 89–95.

Macrae, C. N., Bodenhausen, G. V., & Milne, A. B. (1998). Saying no to unwanted thoughts: Self-focus and the regulation of mental life. *Journal of Personality and Social Psychology*, *74*(3), 578.

Macrae, C. N., Bodenhausen, G. V., Milne, A. B., & Jetten, J. (1994). Out of mind but back in sight: Stereotypes on the rebound. *Journal of Personality and Social Psychology*, *67*(5), 808.

Magura, S., Laudet, A., Mahmood, D., Rosenblum, A., Vogel, H., & Knight, E. (2003). Role of self-help processes in achieving abstinence among dually diagnosed persons. *Addictive Behaviors*, *28*, 399–413.

Maruta, T., Matsumoto, C., & Kanba, S. (2013). Towards the ICD-11: Initiatives taken by the Japanese Society for Psychiatry and Neurology to address needs of patients and clinicians. *Psychiatry and Clinical Neurosciences*, *67*(5), 283–284.

Maruta, T., Volpe, U., Gaebel, W., Matsumoto, C., & Iimori, M. (2014). Should schizophrenia still be named so? *Schizophrenia Research*, *152*(1), 305–306.

Masuda, A., Hayes, S. C., Fletcher, L. B., Seignourel, P. J., Bunting, K., Herbst, S. A., . . . Lillis, J. (2007). Impact of acceptance and commitment therapy versus education on stigma toward people with psychological disorders. *Behaviour Research and Therapy*, *45*(11), 2764–2772.

McCrone, P., Knapp, M., Henri, M., & McDaid, D. (2010). The economic impact of initiatives to reduce stigma: Demonstration of a modelling approach. *Epidemiologia e psichiatria sociale*, *19*(02), 131–139.

McGregor, J. (1993). Effectiveness of role playing and antiracist teaching in reducing student prejudice. *Journal of Educational Research*, *86*(4), 215–226.

Mental Health America. http://www.mentalhealthamerica.net/who-we-are

Meredith, V. M. (2009). Victim identity and respect for human dignity: A terminological analysis. *International Review of the Red Cross*, *91*(874), 259–277.

Merikangas, K., & McClair, V. (2012). Epidemiology of substance use disorders. *Human Genetics*, *131*(6), 779–789. doi:10.1007/s00439-012-1168-0

Minth, H. (2005). The St. Louis Empowerment Center, St. Louis, Missouri. In S. Clay (Ed.), *On our own, together: Peer programs for people with mental illness* (108–122). Nashville, TN: Vanderbilt University Press.

Mojtabai, R., Olfson, M., Sampson, N. A., Jin, R., Druss, B., Wang, P. S., . . . Kessler, R. C. (2011). Barriers to mental health treatment: Results from the National Comorbidity Survey Replication. *Psychological Medicine*, *41*(08), 1751–1761.

Monahan, J., & Arnold, J. (1996). Violence by people with mental illness: A consensus statement by advocates and researchers. *Psychiatric Rehabilitation Journal*, *19*(4), 67.

Morrow D. F. (1996). Coming-out issues for adult lesbians: A group intervention. *Social Work*, *41*(6), 647–656.

Moses, T. (2014). Stigma & family. In Corrigan P. W. (Ed.), *Stigma of disease and disability: Understanding causes and overcoming prejudices* (pp. 247–268). Washington, DC: American Psychological Association.

Mueser, K. T., Glynn, S. M., Corrigan, P. W., & Baber, W. (1996). What's in a name? The preferences of participants in mental health services. *Psychiatric Services*, *47*, 760–761.

Mueser, K. T., Rosenberg, S. D., Goodman, L. A., & Trumbetta, S. L. (2002). Trauma, PTSD, and the course of severe mental illness: An interactive model. *Schizophrenia Research*, *53*(1–2), 123–143. doi:10.1016/S0920-9964(01)00173-6

Narrow, W. E., Regier, D. A., Rae, D. S., Manderscheid, R. W., & Locke, B. Z. (1993). Use of services by persons with mental and addictive disorders: Findings from the National Institute of Mental Health Epidemiologic Catchment Area Program. *Archives of General Psychiatry*, *50*(2), 95–107. doi:10.1001/archpsyc.1993.01820140017002

Nasrallah, H. A. (2009). Medical outcomes from the CATIE schizophrenia study. In J. M. Meyer & H. A. Nasrallah (Eds.). *Medical illness and schizophrenia* (2nd ed., pp. 37–60). Washington, DC: American Psychiatric Publishing Inc.

National Academies of Sciences, Engineering, and Medicine. (2016). *Ending discrimination against people with mental and substance use disorders: The evidence for stigma change*. Washington, DC: National Academies Press.

National Institutes of Health. (2010). *Priorities for the NIH Adherence Research Network*. Retrieved from: https://grants.nih.gov/grants/guide/notice-files/NOT-OD-10-078.html

Nielsen Company. (2009). *A2/M2 Three Screen Report (1st Quarter 2009)*. Retrieved from http://www.nielsen.com/content/dam/corporate/us/en/newswire/uploads/2009/05/nielsen_threescreenreport_q109.pdf

Nieweglowski, K., Corrigan, P. W., Tyas, T., Tooley, A., Dubke, R., Lara, J., . . . Addiction Stigma Research Team. (2017). Exploring the public stigma of substance use disorder through community-based participatory research. *Addiction Research & Theory*, 1–7.

Nyhan, B., Reifler, J., Richey, S., & Freed, G. L. (2014). Effective messages in vaccine promotion: A randomized trial. *Pediatrics*, *133*(4), e835–e842.

Ohayon, M. M. (2000). Prevalence of hallucinations and their pathological associations in the general population. *Psychiatry Research*, *97*(2), 153–164.

Olfson, M., Mojtabai, R., Sampson, N. A., Hwang, I., Druss, B., Wang, P. S., . . . Kessler, R. C. (2009). Dropout from outpatient mental health care in the United States. *Psychiatric Services*, *60*(7), 898–907.

Penn, D. L., & Corrigan, P. W. (2002). The effects of stereotype suppression on psychiatric stigma. *Schizophrenia Research*, *55*, 269–276.

Penn, D. L., & Nowlin-Drummond, A. (2001). Politically correct labels and schizophrenia: A rose by any other name? *Schizophrenia Bulletin*, *27*(2), 197–203.

Pescosolido, B. A., Martin, J. K., Long, J. S., Medina, T. R., Phelan, J. C., & Link, B. G. (2010). "A disease like any other"? A decade of change in public reactions to schizophrenia, depression, and alcohol dependence. *American Journal of Psychiatry*, *167*(11), 1321–1330.

Pew Charitable Trust. (2005). *National reforms needed to help inmates return home*. Retrieved from http://www.pewtrusts.org/en/research-and-analysis/blogs/stateline/2005/01/14/national-reforms-needed-to-help-inmates-return-home

Phelan, J. C., Link, B. G., Stueve, A., & Pescosolido, B. A. (2000). Public conceptions of mental illness in 1950 and 1996: What is mental illness and is it to be feared? *Journal of Health and Social behavior*, *41*(2), 188–207.

Piaget, J. (1985). *The equilibration of cognitive structures: The central problem of intellectual development*. Chicago: University of Chicago Press.

Pincus, F. L. (1999). From individual to structural discrimination. In F. L. Pincus & H. J. Ehrlich (Eds.), *Race and ethnic conflict: Contending views on prejudice, discrimination, and ethnoviolence* (pp. 120–124). Boulder, CO: Westview Press.

Powell, T. (1985). Improving the effectiveness of self-help. *Social Policy, 16*, 22–29.

Rabkin, J. G., Muhlin, G., & Cohen, P. W. (1984). What the neighbors think: Community attitudes toward local psychiatric facilities. *Community Mental Health Journal, 20*(4), 304–312.

Read, J., Haslam, N., Sayce, L., & Davies, E. (2006). Prejudice and schizophrenia: A review of the "mental illness is an illness like any other" approach. *Acta Psychiatrica Scandinavica, 114*(5), 303–318.

Riessman, F. (1965). The "helper" therapy principle. *Social Work, 10*(2), 27–32.

Roberts, L. J., Salem, D., Rappaport, J., Toro, P. A., Luke, D. A., & Seidman, E. (1999). Giving and receiving help: Interpersonal transactions in mutual-help meetings and psychosocial adjustment of members. *American Journal of Community Psychology, 27*, 841–868.

Roe, D. (2001). Progressing from patienthood to personhood across the multidimensional outcomes in schizophrenia and related disorders. *Journal of Nervous and Mental Disease, 189*(10), 691–699.

Rogers, E. S., Chamberlain, J., Ellison, M. L., & Crean, T. (1997). A consumer-constructed scale to measure empowerment among users of mental health services. *Psychiatric Services, 48*(8), 1042–1047

Rosenberg, L. (2013). Mental health stigma overrated? Washington, DC: National Council for Behavior Health. Available at www.thenationalcouncil.org/lindas-corner-office/201307 /is-stigma-overrated-as-a-barrier-to-mental-health-care

Rosenzweig, S. (1936). Some implicit common factors in diverse methods of psychotherapy. *American Journal of Orthopsychiatry, 6*(3), 412–415. http://dx.doi.org/10.1111/j.1939-0025 .1936.tb05248.x

Ruddick, W. (1999). Hope and Deception. *Bioethics, 13*(3–4), 343–357.

Rüsch, N., Corrigan, P. W., Wassel, A., Michaels, P., Larson, J. E., Olschewski, M., . . . Batia, K. (2009a). Self-stigma, group identification, perceived legitimacy of discrimination and mental health service use. *British Journal of Psychiatry, 195*(6), 551–552.

Rüsch, N., Corrigan, P. W., Wassel, A., Michaels, P., Olschewski, M., Wilkniss, S., & Batia, K. (2009b). Ingroup perception and responses to stigma among persons with mental illness. *Acta Psychiatrica Scandinavica, 120*(4), 320–328.

Sartorius, N., Chiu, H., Heok, K. E., Lee, M. S., Ouyang, W. C., Sato, M., . . . Yu, X. (2014). Name change for schizophrenia. *Schizophrenia Bulletin, 40*(2), 255–258.

Sartorius, N., Gaebel, W., Cleveland, H. R., Stuart, H., Akiyama, T., Arboleda-Flórez, J. U. L. I. O., . . . Suzuki, Y. (2010). WPA guidance on how to combat stigmatization of psychiatry and psychiatrists. *World Psychiatry, 9*(3), 131–144.

Satel, S. L. (1998). Are women's health needs really "special"? *Psychiatric Services, 49*(5), 565.

Sayers, J. (2001). The world health report 2001–Mental health: New understanding, new hope. *Bulletin of the World Health Organization, 79*(11), 1085. https://dx.doi.org/10.1590/S0042 -96862001001100014

Schmitt, M. T., Branscombe, N. R., Kobrynowicz, D., & Owen, C. (2002). Perceiving discrimination against one's gender group has different implications for well-being in women and men. *Personality and Social Psychology Bulletin, 28*(2), 197–210.

Schneider, K. (1939). *Psychischer Befund und Psychiatrische Diagnose*. Leipzig: Georg Thieme.

Schomerus, G., Lucht, M., Holzinger, A., Matschinger, H., Carta, M. G., & Angermeyer, M. C. (2011). The stigma of alcohol dependence compared with other mental disorders: A review of population studies. *Alcohol and Alcoholism, 46*(2), 105–112.

Schomerus, G., Schwan, C., & Holzinger, A. (2012). Evolution of public attitudes about mental illness: A systematic review and meta-analysis. *Acta Psychiatrica Scandinavica, 125*, 440–452.

Schulze, B. (2007). Stigma and mental health professionals: A review of the evidence on an intricate relationship. *International Review of Psychiatry, 19*(2), 137–155.

Sears, D. O. (1988). Symbolic racism. In P. A. Katz & D. A. Taylor (Eds.), *Eliminating racism: Profiles in controversy* (pp. 53–84). New York: Plenum Press.

Sells, D., Davidson, L., Jewell, C., Falzer, P., & Rowe, M. (2006). The treatment relationship in peer-based and regular case management for clients with severe mental illness. *Psychiatric Services, 57*, 1179–1184.

Sheehan, L., Fominaya, A. W., Bink, A. B., Kraus, D. J., Schmidt, A., & Corrigan, P. W. (2016). Stigma by any other name. *Psychiatric Services, 67*(12), 1373–1375.

Simon Foundation. (2017, August 3). *Challenge Wall*. Retrieved from http://www.rude2respect .org/join-the-challenge/challenge-wall/

Singer, N. (2009, July 27). Citing risks, lawmakers seek to curb prescription drug commercials. *New York Times*, pp. B1, B6.

Smart, L., & Wegner, D. M. (2000). The hidden costs of hidden stigma. In T. F. Heatherton (Ed.), *The social psychology of stigma* (pp. 220–242). New York: Guilford Press.

Snyder, C., & Rand, K. L. (2003). The case against false hope. *American Psychologist, 58*(10), 820–821. doi:10.1037/0003-066X.58.10.820

Spencer, S. J., Fein, S., Wolfe, C. T., Fong, C., & Dunn, M. A. (1998). Automatic activation of stereotypes: The role of self-image threat. *Personality and Social Psychology Bulletin, 24*(11), 1139–1152.

Spitzer, A., & Cameron, C. (1995). School-age children's perceptions of mental illness. *Western Journal of Nursing Research, 17*(4), 398–415.

Steadman, H. J., Cocozza, J. J., & Melick, M. E. (1978). Explaining the increased arrest rate among mental patients: The changing clientele of state hospitals. *American Journal of Psychiatry, 135*(7), 816-820.

Steele, C. M., & Aronson, J. (1995). Stereotype threat and the intellectual test performance of African Americans. *Journal of Personality and Social Psychology, 69*(5), 797.

Stephan, W. G. (1999). *Reducing prejudice and stereotyping in schools*. New York: Teachers College Press.

Stuart, H., Chen, S. P., Christie, R., Dobson, K., Kirsh, B., Knaak, S., . . . Modgill, G. (2014). Opening minds in Canada: Targeting change. *Canadian Journal of Psychiatry, 59*(1), 13–18.

Substance Abuse and Mental Health Services Administration (SAMHSA). (2013). *Results from the 2012 National Survey on Drug Use and Health: Summary of national findings*. Rockland, MD: Substance Abuse and Mental Health Services Administration.

Tajfel, H. (1981). *Human groups and social categories: Studies in social psychology*. CUP Archive.

Teplin, L. A. (1983). The criminalization of the mentally ill: Speculation in search of data. *Psychological Bulletin, 94*(1), 54.

Teplin, L. A. (1984). Criminalizing mental disorder: The comparative arrest rate of the mentally ill. *American Psychologist, 39*(7), 794.

Torrey, E. F. (2011). Stigma and violence: Isn't it time to connect the dots? *Schizophrenia Bulletin, 37*(5), 892–896.

Townsend, C. (2010). Review of challenges to the human rights of people with intellectual disabilities. *Australian Social Work, 63*(1), 135–136. doi:10.1080/0312407100363II104

Treatment Advocacy Center. (2002). *Approximately 1000 homicides per year in the United States are committed by individuals with severe mental illnesses. Where does this number come from?* [briefing paper]. Retrieved June 17, 2004, from http://www.psychlaws.org/briefingpapers/BP9.htm

University of Indiana. (2002, August 9). *Gauche! Left handers in society.* Retrieved from http://www.indiana.edu/~primate/lspeak2.html#educators

U.S. Census Bureau. (2008). 2008 National Population Projections. Retrieved from www.census.gov/data/tables/2008/demo/popproj/2008-summary-tables.html

Van Gelder, L. (1995, February 14). Howard Geld, 42, advocate for mentally ill, dies. *New York Times.* Retrieved from http://www.nytimes.com/1995/02/14/obituaries/howard-geld-42-advocate-for-mentally-ill-dies.html

Vinacke, W. E. (1949). Stereotyping among national-racial groups in Hawaii: A study in ethnocentrism. *Journal of social psychology, 30*(2), 265–291.

Wahl, O. (1995). *Media madness: Public images of mental illness.* New Brunswick, NJ: Rutgers University Press.

Waite, J., & Easton, A. (2013). *The ECT handbook: The third report of the Royal College of Psychiatrists' Special Committee on ECT.* London: The Royal College of Psiatrists.

Washburn, D. E., Brown, N. L., & Robert, W.A. (1996). *Multicultural education in the United States.* Philadelphia, PA: Inquiry International.

Watson, A. C., Corrigan, P., Larson, J. E., & Sells, M. (2007). Self-stigma in people with mental illness. *Schizophrenia Bulletin, 33*(6), 1312–1318.

Weiner, B. (1995). *Judgments of responsibility: A foundation for a theory of social conduct.* New York: Guilford Press.

Weiner, M. J., & Wright, F. E. (1973). Effects of undergoing arbitrary discrimination upon subsequent attitudes toward a minority group. *Journal of Applied Social Psychology, 3*(1), 94–102.

Werner, S., & Shulman, C. (2015). Does type of disability make a difference in affiliate stigma among family caregivers of individuals with autism, intellectual disability or physical disability? *Journal of Intellectual Disability Research, 59*(3), 272–283.

West, M. L., Yanos, P. T., & Mulay, A. L. (2014). Triple stigma of forensic psychiatric patients: Mental illness, race, and criminal history. *International Journal of Forensic Mental Health, 13*(1), 75–90.

Whitaker, R. (2002). *Mad in America.* New York: Basic Books.

Yanos, P. T., Lucksted, A., Drapalski, A. L., Roe, D., & Lysaker, P. (2015). Interventions targeting mental health self-stigma: A review and comparison. *Psychiatric Rehabilitation Journal, 38*(2), 171.

INDEX

Page numbers followed by f, t, and b refer to figures, tables, and boxes, respectively; those followed by n refer to notes, with note number.